"When Simon Marinker retired from the active practice of surgery in 1987 he had completed 50 years of service to the profession. I had the good fortune to be associated with him for 23 of those years and came to appreciate his concern for the broad subject of the patient's consent to surgery. He was an advocate for full awareness by the patient of the risk-benefit factor in any surgical procedure.

This timely book should be of great benefit, not only to the general public, but to all physicians and surgeons."

Robert G. Martin, M.D., FRCSC, FSOCG
Medical Director
Algoma District Medical Group

Informed Consent to Surgery

Informed Consent to Surgery

**EVERYTHING YOU WANTED TO KNOW ABOUT YOUR
OPERATION BUT WERE AFRAID TO ASK**

by

Simon Marinker, M.D.

Copyright © 1990 by Simon Marinker
First printing October, 1990

All rights reserved. No part of this book may be reproduced in any form by any means without the written permission of the publisher, except by a reviewer, who may quote passages in a review.

Canadian Cataloguing in Publication Data

Marinker, Simon, 1913–
   Informed consent to surgery

   ISBN 0-9694811-0-1
   1. Surgery--Popular works.   2. Informed consent (Medical law)--Canada--Popular works. I. Title.
RD31.3.M37 1990   617   C90-091610-9

Published by **Seldor Publications**
910 - 225 Belleville Street
Victoria, B.C. V8V 4T9

Edited by Elaine Jones.
Cover illustration by Carol Addy, Campaign Communications.
Typesetting by Marian Bantjes, The Typeworks.
Printed and bound in Canada by Hignell Printing, Ltd.

Table of Contents

	ACKNOWLEDGEMENTS	ix
	INTRODUCTION BY DR. S. GORDON FAHRNI	xi
	GENERAL REMARKS ON INFORMED CONSENT	xiii
Chapter 1	PROBLEMS WITH INFORMED CONSENT —SAMPLE CASES	1
Chapter 2	ANESTHESIA	8
Chapter 3	AN OVERALL VIEW OF OPERATIVE COMPLICATIONS	14
Chapter 4	APPENDECTOMY AND HERNIA REPAIRS	26
Chapter 5	OPERATIONS ON THE ESOPHAGUS	31
Chapter 6	OPERATIONS ON THE STOMACH AND SMALL INTESTINE	34
Chapter 7	OPERATIONS ON THE COLON AND RECTUM	40
Chapter 8	OPERATIONS ON THE DIGESTIVE TRACT OF INFANTS	47

Chapter 9	OPERATIONS ON THE BILIARY SYSTEM, PANCREAS AND SPLEEN	52
Chapter 10	THYROID SURGERY AND OTHER TYPES OF NECK SURGERY	60
Chapter 11	OPERATIONS ON THE HEART AND LUNGS	65
Chapter 12	OPERATIONS ON THE ARTERIAL SYSTEM	70
Chapter 13	OTHER OPERATIONS FOR VASCULAR DISORDERS	75
Chapter 14	UROLOGICAL OPERATIONS	81
Chapter 15	SPECIFIC OPERATIONS ON FEMALE PATIENTS	88
Chapter 16	TWO OTHER COMMON OPERATIONS	93
	CONCLUSIONS AND A PERSONAL NOTE BY THE AUTHOR	96
	GLOSSARY OF MEDICAL TERMS	99

ACKNOWLEDGEMENTS

The author wishes to acknowledge, with thanks, the valuable information he has obtained from the professional literature.

The subject of the complications of surgical operations is constantly being updated in the surgical texts and journals, and the following publications, in particular, have been most helpful to the author.

Surgical Clinics of North America. Dec 1983
Edited by Larry C. Carey, M. D.
Published by W. B. Saunders Company

Textbook of Surgery. 1986
Edited by David C. Sabiston Jr., M. D.
Published by W. B. Saunders Company

Principles of Surgery. 1987
Edited by Seymour I. Schwartz, M. D.
Published by McGraw-Hill Book Company

Complications in Surgery and their Management. 1980
Edited by James D. Hardy, M. D.
Published by W. B. Saunders Company

Complications in Surgery and Trauma. 1990
Edited by Lazar J. Greenfield, M. D.
Published by J. B. Lippincott Company

Prognosis of Surgical Disease, 1980
Edited by Ben Eiseman, M. D.
Published by W. B. Saunders Company

Current Surgical Diagnosis and Treatment. 1989
Edited by Lawrence W. Way, M. D.
Published by Appleton and Lange

Last but not least, the author wishes to thank his wife, Maureen, and his daughter, Michele, for their invaluable help and support in the preparation of this book.

Introduction

By Dr. Gordon S. Fahrni

I first met Simon Marinker about 1943 when he was serving as a young surgeon in an army hospital in Regina, Saskatchewan, with the rank of Captain. As consulting surgeon in the RCAMC, it was part of my job to provide a competent surgical staff for army hospitals.

Dr. Marinker's qualifications were such that he was sent to head up the surgical service in one of our largest Canadian Military Training Centres in Dundurn, Saskatchewan.

When the war of 1939–45 was over, he established a surgical practice in Victoria, B.C. In his retirement, fortunately for us all, he has written this book on a subject that has become an increasingly prominent feature in the lawsuits for malpractice.

This book has gone into great detail on the complications of most of the common surgical operations in a very comprehensive manner. It must always be remembered that these complications are comparatively rare but, nevertheless, possible.

It is a book that will serve people who become worried and apprehensive about a proposed operation. The danger of such aprehension is that the patient will magnify and put these seldom seen complications into the wrong perspective. This attitude may result in the refusal of a badly needed operation or submission to surgery with an unhappy and fearful attitude. No surgeon wants to operate on such a patient.

The ideal mental attitude is one of confidence in your surgeon, as it is his or her job to do everything possible to bring about a completely satisfactory operative procedure.

This book will also serve the need of surgeons.

I congratulate the author on producing a comprehensive book on a subject that has become important in these changing social times.

Gordon S. Fahrni, MD, FRCS(C), FACS, DABS, FICS (Hon.), is past president of the Canadian Medical Association and the acknowledged elder statesman of Canadian Surgery.

General Remarks on Informed Consent

What, precisely, is meant by informed consent? It means that you, the patient, accept a particular line of investigation and treatment based on the information you receive from your doctors. If your problem involves surgery, you will get this information from your family doctor, your surgeon, and others who will be managing your treatment.

Informed consent also means that you understand the proposed investigation and treatment of your condition, the goals of that treatment, and the possible risks,—and it means that these requirements are fulfilled prior to the commencement of investigation and treatment. It also means that you have been informed about alternative methods of treatment.

As far as this book is concerned, the discussion of these matters will be confined to common surgical operations and their possible complications. The book also includes a glossary of medical terms used in the text.

The laws that govern what is legally designated "Informed Consent" are both confused and contradictory, but there are certain basic principles. You, the patient, have the right to be given an explanation of the proposed surgery, and of the possible risks; these include the risks of the investigations, the anesthetic, the operation and the postoperative recovery period. You also have the right to refuse any portion of these explanations, particularly when it comes to the unpleasant subject of complications, both during and following surgery. In the past, most patients didn't want to know about surgical risks, but with each new generatiom more and more patients do want to know before making up their minds.

The effectiveness of the explanation depends on the ability of your physician and your surgeon to give simple descriptions in simplified language, and on your ability to absorb the information and to understand it clearly. How much you remember about this information, both before and after the operation, is extremely variable. Is there a safeguard to make sure that you both understand and remember?

In the field of medical drugs there is an excellent book entitled *Understanding Canadian Prescription Drugs* by Dorothy L.Smith, Pharm.D. published by Key Porter Books. It lists the majority of prescription drugs, the indications for their use, the contraindications, and the adverse side effects. There are also excellent books for the public on the subject of surgical operations, written in understandable terms, but no such book—of which the author is aware—that lists the complications of the common surgical operations and is written specifically for the surgical patient.

This book addresses a wide range of the major surgical operations— the most common ones—and their complications. No attempt is made to give statistical odds for any of these complications in any particular patient, as these are affected by the individual's physical and mental condition prior to surgery, by the personal and past history, and by known or hidden genetic factors.

The facilities of the particular hospital, the experience of the surgical team and dozens of other factors may affect the outcome of the procedure. What is the status and safety of the operating room (OR) equipment? Did your anesthetist quarrel with spouse or children prior to surgery. Did your surgeon have a good night's sleep or stay awake, worrying about a tough case or some bad news from the income tax department? Are the nurses involved in bitter contract negotiations? Is any or all of the operation done by someone other than your designated surgeon? How good is the cardiac resuscitation team, the intensive care unit, the standard surgical ward care? These are all possible factors which may affect the incidence of complications in any individual case, but do not enter into calculations of national statistics.

General Remarks xv

Other items of importance in discussing risks with your doctors are the alternative methods of managing your problem, both operative and nonoperative, and the risks of refusing the proposed surgery. For example, if you have acute appendicitis and refuse an operation, you may die of peritonitis. In this case the **known** risks of refusing surgery far outweigh the **possible** risks of the surgery itself.

While this reference book has been written to inform patients of the possible surgical complications, it should be remembered that **most of these risks are preventable.**

A considerable degree of prevention is in your hands if you have been booked for elective surgery, with a waiting list of weeks or months. You can stop smoking or at least cut down on a steady basis, do some deep breathing and effective coughing exercises on a daily basis, eat a balanced diet and follow a regular exercise program, including a daily walk. If you are taking any medications, make sure your doctors are fully aware of them, especially those you have been getting "across the counter." If you are a heavy drinker, start cutting down day by day. Above all, seek your doctors' guidance in taking the necessary steps to make you safe for the planned surgery. They, in turn, will do everything possible to make the surgery safe for you.

With the overall high standards of surgical care now available from coast to coast, the incidence of most of these complications is gratifyingly low and steadily diminishing. They do exist, however, just as the risks of driving to work, crossing the road, living with polluted air, earth and water, are those we knowingly face each day in modern society. It is the sacred duty of your surgeon and of the medical profession as a whole to make every effort to reduce the incidence of these complications. Nevertheless, they may occur even when your surgeon is highly skilled and has taken every possible precaution to prevent mishap.

According to the laws governing informed consent, however, your surgeon will be adjudged guilty of negligence if it is ruled that he or she failed to give you the necessary information to obtain such informed consent. It is therefore in your surgeon's interest as well as yours that you be fully aware of all the above considerations before you consent to your operation.

This book has been written to aid both you and your doctors, and to avoid confusion and injustice. It is meant to be used as a reference book, but with the warning that you should clear up any remaining points of concern with your surgeon and personal physician prior to giving written consent.

CHAPTER 1

Problems with the Consent Process—Sample Cases

James Scott, aged twenty-six, was a basically healthy bank teller with a medical history that was essentially negative prior to his attack of suspected acute appendicitis. The only positive items in his past history were an allergy to sulfa drugs, severe heartburn whenever he took aspirin, and the usual childhood fevers. He was on no medications, was a nonsmoker, and took only an occasional drink of scotch or a beer. He was fond of sports, especially badminton, and there was no cancer, diabetes, heart trouble, high blood pressure, kidney or lung disease in his family history.

At 6.30 p.m on the day prior to his admission to hospital, he had dinner at home with his wife and young daughter. The dinner consisted of a salad including crisp lettuce, tomato, cucumber and roquefort dressing, followed by roast chicken and french fried potatoes. He had coffee but no dessert; he was trying to avoid gaining weight, which had remained steady at about 170 pounds for the past 2-3 years and which he felt was just about right for his height of 6 feet.

At 1 a.m. he was awakened with cramps across his mid-abdomen, which became quite severe and were accompanied by nausea and vomiting: he brought up most of what he had eaten, but with no relief. While in the bathroom he tried to pass gas or have a bowel movement, but was unsuccessful.

When examined at the hospital emergency department the following morning at 10 a.m., the pain was much sharper and seemed to be located in the lower right belly, although he still had occasional general-

2   Informed Consent to Surgery

ized cramps. He was still nauseated and had no appetite for food. His temperature was slightly raised, his pulse rate was slightly fast but regular, and his blood pressure was normal. Significant findings were restricted to his abdomen, where there was tenderness and muscular stiffening in the right lower area. There was also pain when the examiner suddenly released the pressure of his examining hand. This was recorded on the emergency chart as "rebound positive." The abdominal sounds as determined with the stethoscope were recorded as "peristalsis minus," (a diminution of the bowel sounds) and rectal examination was negative. The blood count was consistent with an acute inflammatory condition and the urine sample was entirely normal. (The word "acute", used medically, means of sudden or rapid onset).

These findings were considered to be compatible with a diagnosis of acute appendicitis and there was nothing in the abdominal and chest X-rays to indicate any other diagnosis. At this point the staff surgeon on emergency call was summoned by the emergency resident and reexamined the patient. She, too, diagnosed acute appendicitis and recommended to the patient and his wife that an operation to remove the inflamed appendix should be done as soon as possible, as delay would increase the chances of peritonitis (a dangerous infection of the abdominal cavity) due to ruptured appendicitis.

At operation, the appendix was found to be entirely normal and this was confirmed by microscopic exmination of the removed organ. There were no other positive findings in the abdomen and the diagnosis was provisionally changed to bacterial gastroenteritis; in fact, two days later the patient began to develop diarrhea with frequent loose, blood-stained stools. This cleared up slowly with intravenous fluids and suitable antibiotics against what proved to be salmonella infection.

The patient remained lethargic and weak and his diarrhea gradually responded to Imodium tablets. Unfortunately he developed phlebitis in his legs and, despite the immediate administration of vigorous anticlotting therapy, James Scott died suddenly at 4 a.m. on the sixth postoperative day, due to massive "pulmonary embolism." This was less than twelve hours after the first appearance of the phlebitis. At the autopsy it was concluded that the phlebitis probably developed insidiously for several days postoperatively with no symptoms. The condition had then progressed just as insidiously up the venous system, with a massive blood clot becoming loosened and lodging in the major vessels of the lungs.

The surgeon and hospital were sued by the Scott family. The main point of the plaintiff's contention was that at no time was the complication of blood clots in the lungs discussed with the patient prior to surgery, the patient's wife having been present at both examinations and attendant discussions. Since the surgery had proven unnecessary because of the mistaken diagnosis, the fatal complication that had never been mentioned need never have occurred.

Bessie Lufkind, aged fifty-eight, was chief cook at a restaurant.

For five days prior to her hospital admission, she had been off work and home in bed because of severe abdominal pains going up to the lower right chest and through to the back. At the same time she noticed that her eyes and skin were turning yellow, her urine was getting very dark and her bowel movements were a strange greyish colour. Since she had experienced similar but less severe attacks in the past, for which she had taken some pain pills, she simply stayed in bed and took more and more pills until she got no relief at all.

When questioned in the emergency department, on admission by ambulance, it was discovered that she had lived alone for the past seven years following the death of her husband. She said that she stayed away from doctors because they urged her to reduce (she had always been overweight and hadn't been below 200 lbs for at least ten years, despite being only 5 ft 4 in height).

The doctors also wanted her to quit smoking, because of her persistent cough with considerable phlegm, and her shortness of breath. As if that weren't bad enough, they usually discovered her alcoholic habit and wished to deprive her of one of her few remaining comforts. As for food, her appetite had always been unrelenting until this recent illness.

Further enquiry revealed the fact that she had a clear-cut history of recurrent heart failure, bronchitis and emphysema, and mild diabetes which had been inadequately treated. The family history included heart disease on both sides of the family, as well as diabetes, obesity and high blood pressure. The most important feature of the patient's background was the degree of self-neglect and her failure to keep the appointments with her physician, or to accept medical advice and treatment.

Fortunately, on this occasion, her oldest daughter and son-in-law had come to visit her from across town and discovered how ill she was. They called an ambulance despite her loud protestations and accompanied her to the hospital, where they were able to fill in many of the medical facts of the patient's past which she had tried to conceal.

A definitive diagnosis was soon made: "Gallstones, with obstruction of the common bile duct producing an increasing obstructive jaundice, with evidence of early liver failure." This diagnosis was fully substantiated by ultrasound examination of the abdomen, which showed stones in the gallbladder and obstructing a distended common bile duct. The lab results revealed a moderate anemia, a marked increase of bile pigments in the blood, and evidence of liver impairment. The blood sugar was raised and both sugar and bile pigments were present in the urine. Other findings during the routine physical examination showed enlargement of the heart and irregularity of the pulse, high blood pressure, the presence of severe emphysema, and advanced varicose veins of both legs with evidence of previous deep vein phlebitis.

The attending surgeon informed the patient, in the presence of her daughter and son-in-law, of his findings and diagnosis. He strongly advised an operation to remove the gallbladder and stones and to relieve the obstruction of the bile duct. The patient was told that the risks of postoperative lung complications were considerable, as were problems with her diseased heart, diabetes, and diseased veins. He also stated that these risks were compounded by her severe obesity, smoking, and fondness for alcohol. **Her only chance for survival, however, lay with corrective surgery,** and this point was fully stressed.

At this juncture Mrs. Lufkind refused to accept the proposed operation and remained quite adamant, despite all arguments and explanations. Eight days later she died of liver failure complicated by massive pneumonia.

The surgeon and the hospital were sued by the family on a charge of scaring the patient to such a degree that she was irrevocably terrified of dying following surgery.

These two cases are fictitious, but they are based on the writer's experience in all aspects of general surgery over a period of fifty years, and are composites of actual cases he has known about during that time. They indicate the difficulties of what the lawyers call "Informed Consent", a term which is a gross misnomer in many important respects.

It is easy enough for a surgeon to "grandstand" and pretend to the patient and the patient's family, probably even to himself or herself, that the listener is able to hear, comprehend, recall, evaluate and accept the information—both intellectually and emotionally—without confusion, terror or false confidence. It is equally easy for the patient to fool himself or herself into thinking he or she is informed, or even to avoid the whole issue because of being too frightened to think about it.

Every surgical operation, whether performed in a major operating room or in a minor surgical facility such as an emergency or outpatient department, carries a risk of complications. If such unfortunate results follow surgery for a life-threatening condition, they will carry less upsetting or tragic impact than with surgery for less serious conditions. Such unfortunate results may have nothing to do with the calibre of care given by the surgical team, but they may, nonetheless, be a basis for litigation by the patient or patient's family.

As far as the plaintiff's lawyer is concerned, the level of professional care may or may not be a factor in involving the doctors and hospital in a lawsuit. The more difficult it is to find genuine medical mismanagement, incompetence or negligence, the more likely it becomes that the major charge will be a lack of informed consent.

Let us return to our two composite cases. Should Mr. Scott have been told about the possibility of pulmonary embolism? Some would say "Absolutely!", others would say "Never!", and most would say "I'm not sure." Legally, of course, the answer is "Absolutely" but then lawyers are not good surgeons, even if they happen to be good lawyers.

6   *Informed Consent to Surgery*

In the case of Mrs. Lufkind the surgeon would win the approval of lawyers for the high level of information given the patient, but that same information frightened the patient away from what might have been life-saving surgery.

It is important for patients to keep things in perspective when assessing information necessary for informed consent. Every beneficial medication may have adverse side-effects: this comes under the heading of the "risk-benefit" factor. In the same way, every surgical procedure is evaluated by the referring physician, the anesthetist, and the surgeon on the basis of this risk- benefit factor. The anticipated benefits of the proposed surgery are balanced against the anticipated risks. The benefits might be the saving of a life, the cure of a severe surgical disease, palliation, or simply cosmetic improvement, while the risks vary according to the patient's general condition at the time of surgery as well as the surgeon's record of complications and mortality for the specific operation. These factors are often far more important in assessing the actual chances of complications or mortality than can be gauged by a routine recitation of possible risks.

Perhaps the most important step that a patient can take prior to facing surgery is to find out as much as possible about his or her surgeon. This is not too easy at the present time, and perhaps in some future utopian era of the health-care system it may be possible to obtain a professional rating of surgeons, to include competence, integrity, experience, and record of operative and postoperative mortality and complications.

This can be estimated—at present—within the hospital establishment by obtaining an evaluation from his or her fellow-surgeons, and even more objectively from the anesthetists, pathologists, and radiologists who know the surgeon's work; unfortunately this "inside" information is rarely available to the patient.

Finally, we must consider the wide disparity between surgeons in what they believe should or should not be told to the patient, and what is or is not important for the patient to know about the proposed surgery. A second surgical opinion could be helpful in establishing a superior rapport but, conversely, the second surgeon could prove to be simply more persuasive or glib rather than more competent.

The hospital setting must also be considered. Should most major surgery be done in university-related teaching hospitals? The large majority of major surgical operations can be handled safely and competently in nonteaching hospitals, and too much centralization of surgical facilities in a country the size of Canada, or the U.S.A., may not be in the best interest of the patient. It often proves a hardship to the patient's family.

Some of our finest surgeons practice in nonteaching hospitals, and it should be remembered that talent should never be measured geographically. In fact, the death rates, complication rates and cure rates in community hospitals compare favourably with those in the major university centres. The number of surgical specialists and subspecialists constantly moving into smaller communities can only improve the overall standard of care and reduce the unnecessary costs of overcentralization.

The author has attempted in the past to get various official medical organizations to publish a list of common surgical operations, with appropriate explanations and descriptions of complications, in the same way that the pharmaceutical compendiums list and explain the drugs and their adverse effects.

This book attempts to set forth as simply as possible the common operations in surgery and the recognized possible complications which may occur during and following surgery, of which the most important and irreversible is death.

Since the risks of operative surgery commence with those of anesthesia, these will be considered first.

CHAPTER 2

Anesthesia

The term "anesthesia" means the absence of sensation and, in the context of this chapter, refers mainly to the absence of pain.

General anesthesia is essentially produced by the inhalation of special gases which cause total loss of consciousness. Of course, even with regional (nerve-block) anesthesia, intravenous regional anethesia, spinal, epidural and local infiltration anesthesia, the patient may be put to sleep by the intravenous injection of a potent tranquilizer. Modern anesthesiology is a highly skilled specialty, and it has advanced in complexity and excellence over the past few decades at an incredible rate.

The broad heading of anesthesia includes:
1. General anesthesia.
2. Regional anesthesia by nerve-block.
3. Intravenous regional anesthesia.
4. Spinal and epidural anesthesia.
5. Local anesthesia (soft tissue infiltration).

General Anesthesia Before considering general anesthesia, a brief review of the respiratory system is in order. Air is breathed in through the nose or mouth and proceeds into the *pharynx*, which is the cavity between the nose and mouth above and the *larynx*, or voice box, below. The air proceeds down the *trachea*, or windpipe, and this in turn divides into right and left channels known as the primary bronchi (plural of bronchus). These further subdivide into secondary *bronchi*, and then into the smaller air tubes, called bronchioles. Finally, these *bronchioles* communicate with the tiny air-sacs of the lung, known as *alveoli*.

General anesthesia is administered after premedicating the patient with a drug such as atropine to dry up the natural secretions in the mouth, nose, throat, bronchial passages and lungs, and a narcotic such as Demerol (pethidine) to make the patient drowsy. The patient then receives a dose of Pentothal or a similar tranquilizing drug intravenously, combined with a muscular relaxant such as those of the curare series. Next, a cuffed tube is passed down the trachea, thus obtaining a "closed" anesthetic system for the inhalation of anesthetic gases in combination with an adequate level of oxygen. **In the main, modern anesthesia is safe and dependable**, but the following is a simplified list of what can go wrong under the worst of circumstances.

Complications

- Drug Reactions
  The patient may have an allergy, an intolerance or an idiosyncrasy towards any of the drugs under anesthesia.
- Technical Difficulties
  There may be difficulties in finding a suitable vein or difficulties in passing the (*endotracheal*) tube into a distorted or constricted airway.
- Gas Machine Problems
  There may be hidden leaks in the gas system or faulty connections, and the flowmeters may be giving incorrect and misleading readings.
- Prior Medications
  Drugs taken by the patient prior to operation, either self-administered or prescribed by a physician, may interfere with the premedication drugs or the anesthetic components themselves, and sometimes to a highly dangerous degree. This interference may act to increase or decrease the actions of the anesthetic agents, and the use of such drugs by the patient prior to surgery is often not disclosed to the anesthetist.
- Injection Mishaps
  Accidental injection of induction drugs such as pentothal into an artery instead of a vein can result in loss of a portion of the involved limb, such as the forearm and hand, due to progressive gangrene. On rare occasions, even permanent nerve damage may occur in a similar manner.

- Problems with Passage of the *Endotracheal Tube*
  Injury to the mouth, teeth, dental appliances, throat, or upper respiratory passages, may occur with passage of the tube into the trachea, especially if passage of the tube runs into unexpected difficulties.
- Genetically Related Problems
  In certain patients with a specific genetic defect, one of the commonly used muscle relaxants which is generally employed with safety during general anesthesia cannot be properly metabolized, and causes a prolonged period of general paralysis. Another complication of general anesthesia which has a genetic basis is *malignant hyperthermia*, a condition that is extremely rare but carries a mortality of over 25 percent even with the best possible emergency treatment. It, too, has a metabolic basis and is characterized by muscular rigidity and a rapid rise of temperature to extraordinary levels, leading to death, or to blood disorders, permanent neurological damage and other adverse conditions.
- Improper Positioning
  This may occur with the unconscious patient and lead to nerve damage in a limb that is subjected to undue pressure or stretch. Over 10 percent of all reported nerve paralyses in the limbs have been caused by incorrect positioning of the unconscious patient.
- Respiratory Problems
  During Recovery In the recovery phase from general anesthetics there may be respiratory complications such as lung collapse, retention of mucus in the lungs, and pneumonia.
- Aspiration
  There may also be complications due to regurgitation of stomach contents into the throat and inhalation into the lungs.
- Toxicity
  Finally, there may be complications due to toxic effects of the anesthetic gases themselves, with damage to the liver or kidneys.

REGIONAL NERVE BLOCK

This entails injection of local anesthetics around nerves which supply the region to be anesthetized.

Complications

- Injuries
  This method carries a low complication rate, except for the possibility of injury to one or more nerves or to an artery that is in the vicinity of the injection.

INTRAVENOUS REGIONAL ANESTHESIA

This is performed by injecting a local anesthetic agent into a limb-vein which has been carefully isolated from the general circulation by special tourniquet control.

Complications

- Dispersal into the General Blood Stream
  Escape of the agent into the circulation may occur due to faulty tourniquet control or by the sudden release of the agent out of the limb when the cuff is deflated. This may produce mild to severe toxic systemic symptoms, and certain anesthetic agents may produce phlebitis, neuritis or paralysis.

SPINAL ANESTHESIA

This entails the injection of local anesthetic into the fluid space surrounding the spinal cord.

Complications

- Backache
  The complications following spinal anesthesia are far from unknown. The most obvious is backache, which may be temporary or long-lasting.
- Infection
  This is in the form of *spinal meningitis*. Fortunately it is rare, and should not occur with a sterile technique.
- Noninfective Meningitis
  A serious chronic inflammation of the spinal membranes, that is not due to bacterial infection, may occur as a result of chemical contaminants introduced into the vertebral canal.

12   Informed Consent to Surgery

- Headache
  This symptom, of varying persistence, occurs in an appreciable proportion of patients having spinal anesthesia, especially when larger needles are used.
- Permanent Nerve Damage
  This occurs in about one in five thousand patients who have had spinal anesthesia.
- Respiratory Complications
  These may occur if the level of spinal blockade is too high and involves the nerves of the rib cage.

EPIDURAL ANESTHESIA

Unlike spinal anesthesia, epidural anesthesia involves a spinal injection of the chemical agent just outside the main fluid space around the spinal cord.

Complications

- Injuries
  Nerve and bloodvessel tissues in the epidural space may be injured, or the needle may accidentally enter the fluid space and the procedure has to be aborted.
- Infection Abscess
  formation may occur, and most of the recorded septic complications are commoner with the use of an indwelling catheter that is left in place for a period of time.

LOCAL ANESTHETICS

These are anesthetic solutions injected into the soft tissues.

Complications

- Allergy
  Local anesthetics may produce allergic reactions, and in a patient with an unrecorded allergy to "caine" drugs such as novocaine, pontocaine, benzocaine, and cocaine, the reaction may be *anaphylactic*, with cardiovascular collapse, swelling of the larynx, and generalized hives on the skin.

- Toxicity
  On the other hand the anesthetic agents may cause toxic reactions that are not allergic and are related to dosage.
  These may include tingling in the face, ringing in the ears, convulsions, respiratory and cardiovascular depression and even cardiac arrest.
- Injection Mishaps
  Accidental injection of local anesthetic solutions into a blood vessel instead of soft tissues will increase the chances of such complications as allergic or toxic reactions during local infiltration anesthesia.

CHAPTER 3

An Overall View of Operative Complications

Most operations commence with a skin incision. Next, the underlying fat is incised, and then the muscles are either incised or separated. In dividing the subcutaneous fat there may be bleeding from the small blood vessels; these may be dealt with by applying fine artery forceps to the bleeding points and then tying with fine ligatures. Alternatively, a cautery (a heated point—usually by electrical current) may be used to seal off small bleeding points or to cut muscles (by means of a cautery-blade) and other tissues with less bleeding. Middle sized vessels may be ligated or sealed with special clips which can be applied with special forceps, especially in deep and difficult locations. The largest vessels may require delicate suturing in order to close a major hole in the vessel wall.

BLEEDING

Bleeding at surgery can be mild, significant, severe, or catastrophic. Mild bleeding is usually from capillaries and very small veins. Significant bleeding is from small arteries or larger veins, and severe or catastrophic bleeding is from major blood vessels.

The amount of bleeding will be influenced by interference with the clotting mechanism, as in defects such as hemophilia, and other blood disorders such as leukemias and disorders of the spleen and liver. In some patients who have been on anticlotting medications, bleeding may be increased, and aspirin is a common culprit.

Complications

- Massive Bleeding
  When this cannot rapidly be brought under control may prove fatal, or may produce the condition of *surgical shock*, with a fall in blood pressure and *cardiovascular* collapse.
- Compression
  A collection of blood inside the closed cranial cavity may cause pressure on the brain, with resultant paralysis or death. A collection of blood in the chest may compress the lung. A collection of blood in the abdomen may cause paralysis of the intestines.
- *Hematoma*
  This is a collection of blood in the soft tissues and may be fluid or clotted. If it occurs in a closed muscle compartment it may damage the muscles or nerves in that space, and any swelling in such a compartment can cause death of the muscle by pressure which shuts off the blood supply. Any blood collection is extremely vulnerable to infection and should therefore be drained off as early as possible, quite aside from the other reasons for such drainage.

INFECTION

Any part of the body may be invaded by bacteria. This results in the production of a solid swelling of the soft tissues, called *cellulitis*, a fluid collection of pus, called an *abscess*, or involvement of the lining membranes of body cavities. In the abdomen this is called *peritonitis*, in the chest it is called empyema, in the spinal canal and brain membranes it is called *meningitis*. If the bacteria invade the blood stream the condition is known as *bacteremia*, and if they multiply there it is called *septicemia*.

As a surgical complication, infection may result from operating in an infected or dirty field, such as operating on the colon or in a severely contaminated road-accident case. It may also occur if there is a major breach of stringent antiseptic and aseptic techniques in the operating room. Harmful bacteria may proliferate where the choice of antibiotics is incorrect, where they haven't been employed, or where the dosage is inadequate.

An intermediate phase between local and bloodborne infection is an inflammation of the lymphatic vessels causing red streaks up the limb,

16   *Informed Consent to Surgery*

and arrest of the infection at the lymph nodes, which become swollen and painful, typically in the neck, axilla, and groin.

The bacteria which cause infection are of two main groups: *aerobic* which require oxygen, and *anaerobic* which thrive in the absence of oxygen.

SPECIFIC INFECTIVE COMPLICATIONS

- *Symbiotic Gangrene*
  Sometimes a deadly combination of bacterial types in an operative wound can cause this condition, a progressive destruction of skin and deeper soft tissues which is extremely difficult to manage.
- *Tetanus* (Lockjaw)
  This is a rare type of anaerobic operative infection in elective surgery. Tetanus occurring in patients with contaminated wounds resulting from accidents, however, is a well-known hazard.
- *Gas Gangrene*
  This is another dreaded anaerobic infection which may occur in muscle wounds, such as in compound fractures in which dirt, foreign material and dead tissue may be present.
- *Necrosis*
  This is the medical term for death of tissues. It may occur due to direct injury, loss of blood-supply, sutures that are too constricting, or bacterial and other microbial infection.
- Fungal Infections
  These may be seen in patients who have received large doses of "broad spectrum antibiotics" which kill a wide range of bacteria, including the beneficial ones in the intestinal tract. This results in an overgrowth of fungi, especially the one known as *candida albicans*, and the infection may spread through the bloodstream. The infection may enter via a bladder catheter, or via an indwelling feeding catheter in a major vein.

Each and every surgical operation may be followed by infection; the mild infections are easy to manage, the severe ones may be life-threatening.

RESPIRATORY PROBLEMS

This group of postoperative complications may be related to preoperative factors, to anesthetic and drug factors, and to operative factors. The immediate causes are increased bronchial secretions, undue viscosity of these secretions, reduced coughing reflex, reduced respiratory effort and efficiency, including automatic sighing and yawning, and impaired movement of the chest and abdominal muscles and the diaphragm.

- Gastric Tube Problems
  The prolonged presence of an indwelling gastric suction tube inserted via the nasal passages can injure the larynx, increase nasopharyngeal and bronchial secretions and thus increase the likelihood of respiratory complications, especially in the debilitated and aged patient.
- Pain
  In the early postoperative period, wound-related pain may be the cause of respiratory inhibitions, especially in operations on the upper abdomen and chest.
- Pre-existing Chronic Lung Disease
  Such conditions as bronchitis and emphysema may cause increased bronchial secretions and dehydration may cause increased mucus viscosity.
- Immobility
  Failure to move adequately and to change position frequently may be contributory factors, and narcotic drugs to relieve pain may dull the respiratory reflexes.
- Cigarette Smoking
  This is a notorious factor in increasing the frequency and degree of respiratory complications.
- Excessive or Inadequate Weight
  Another preoperative factor of considerable importance is obesity and, conversely, still another is debility.
- Lung Collapse
  The actual lung conditions which may occur postoperatively are collapse of one or both lungs, pneumonia and abscess.
  Lung collapse, called *atelectasis*, may involve only very small segments of one or both lungs (extremely frequent), one or more lobes of the lung, or one or both entire lungs—much less common but life-threatening.
- Pneumonia
  In the postoperative period this occurs mainly as a result of lung collapse when bacteria invade the collapsed pulmonary areas.

18   *Informed Consent to Surgery*

- Aspiration
  Another cause of pneumonia is the inhalation of regurgitated stomach contents by the anesthetized, narcotized, or debilitated patient. This is called *aspiration pneumonia*.
  Lung abscesses are usually caused by the inhalation of infected material, especially after teeth extractions and removal of tonsils.
- *Acute (Adult) Respiratory Distress Syndrome (ARDS)*
  This is a special type of respiratory complication that has become increasingly identified over recent decades. It may occur in massively injured patients and is then usually called *shock lung*. It may result from overinfusion of intravenous fluids or overtransfusion of blood in the patient's treatment. (A *syndrome* is a group of symptoms and clinical signs that are characteristic of a particular condition).
- *Sepsis*
  This may be either in the form of infection in the lung or septicemia from infection in another area, and is another important contributory factor in ARDS.
- *Pulmonary Edema*
  Excessive fluid retention in the lung is usually secondary to cardiac failure or inadequate oxygen intake.
- *Fat Embolism*
  This is a condition in which globules escape into the bloodstream from the exposed bone marrow and lodge in various parts of the body, and may occur in severe fracture cases.
  The most important of these locations are the lungs and the brain. In the lungs, the effects are very similar to those of pulmonary edema.

These respiratory complications are extremely frequent and of the utmost importance. They may be minimized to a significant degree in non-emergency situations by a program of preoperative education and preparation of the patient, and postoperatively by the patient's courage and determination.

Once again, it should be emphasized that most of these complications can be avoided by appropriate preventive measures and, when they occur, most can be cured or ameliorated by correct treatment.

DIGESTIVE COMPLICATIONS

- *Parotitis*
  Extreme dryness of the mouth may be due to the use of atropine and

similar drugs. In debilitated patients and those with dental sepsis this may lead to a dangerous condition known as *acute postoperative parotitis*, and is due to infection, cellulitis and abscess formation in the same salivary gland that is involved in the viral condition of mumps (the *parotid* gland).
- Sore Throat and Swallowing Difficulties
  These may be the after-effect of anesthetic intubation.
  Nausea and vomiting are a frequent after-effect of general anesthesia. Regurgitation of stomach contents is more likely to occur in patients who have a history of this condition prior to surgery.
- Gastric Retention and Distention
  These may occur postoperatively and are commoner in patients with a history of ulcer or gastritis.
- Inhibition of Intestinal Motility
  This is quite common following general anesthesia and following abdominal procedures. In the more severe degrees of this condition, with gross distension and failure to pass gas, it is known as *paralytic ileus* and may be an indication of peritonitis.
- Postoperative Constipation
  This is common and easily combatted with an appropriate dietary intake and a daily bowel routine. Painful prolapsing hemorrhoids can occur with enemas and excessive straining at stool. Like the other gastrointestinal problems in the postoperative patient they are easily managed.
- Bladder Problems
  Urinary retention is much commoner in men and especially in those with enlargement of the prostate. An early trip to the privacy of a bathroom rather than the use of a bottle in bed may be the best antidote.
- Blood Clots
  Postoperative clotting of blood in a bloodvessel, usually one of the leg veins, is known as *thrombosis*. The danger lies in the clot extending up the vessel, then finally breaking off and lodging in the lungs: this dread complication, often fatal, is known as *pulmonary embolism*. Both of these conditions can often be anticipated, especially in high-risk patients, and appropriate measures of prevention and therapy can be undertaken. These include a weight-reduction program for the obese if time permits, avoidance of bed rest, increased mobilization, and the administration of controlled anticlotting agents—commencing shortly before surgery.

WOUND COMPLICATIONS

Wound healing is an incredibly complex microscopic and chemical process and is influenced by many factors. These include nutritional factors, particularly proteins and Vitamin C, trapped blood or serum in the wound, and infection.

- Operative Factors
  These include the type of sutures that are used, absorbable or nonabsorbable, mono- or multifilament, light or heavy, biological or synthetic, metallic wire, staples or clips, skin-tapes or some of the new biocompatible tissue glues.
- Technical Defects
  Too many sutures may interfere with wound-repair as much as too few sutures, and tying the sutures too tightly is just as harmful as tying them too loosely.
- Rapid or Slow Surgery
  Fast surgery may lead to rough handling of the tissues and impair wound repair, but slow surgery may lead to increased drying of the tissues and the chance of infection with similar impairment of wound healing.
- The Administration of Steroids (Cortisone Drugs)
  When given to the surgical patient before, during, or after operation, they may impair wound healing. The same is true of many of the anticancer drugs that are in common use today and those immunity-suppressing drugs employed in transplant surgery.
- Diabetes
  Diabetic patients heal poorly and are prone to infection.
- Previous Radiation of the Wound Area (for Cancer Therapy)
  This may also inhibit healing.
- Wound Disruption (Wide Separation)
  When this occurs following major abdominal surgery (as in the nonfatal complication of "burst abdomen") it may be accompanied by evisceration of the intestines. This complication is commoner with vertical than with horizontal abdominal incisions, and is commoner in patients with persistent distension, retching, obesity, or debility.
  Patients with asthma and other respiratory problems are also at increased risk of this complication, because of unremitting attacks of coughing.
- Infection of the Wound
  This may produce a wound abscess, tissue destruction, or nonheal-

ing. If nonabsorbable sutures are involved, stitch abscesses may develop either at the skin level or at deeper levels, with the formation of *suture sinuses* (septic tunnels that discharge pus). They lead from buried suture material to the skin and are commoner with multi-strand sutures and large knots. Wound infection is the most potent enemy of smooth repair of wounds and increases the amount of pain and tenderness in the incision. The moment any postoperative patient exhibits a fever, wound infection should be the prime suspect.

- Unsatisfactory Scars

  Woundscars may become contracted, hypertrophic, or *keloid*, with ugly hard ridges replacing the smooth fine line of a well-healed incision. These are annoying cosmetic results and are serious to the patient whose beauty is paramount, but sometimes keloids are unpreventable and often difficult to cure, although some degree of spontaneous improvement may occur with the passage of time.

- Hernias

  These may occur following any previous abdominal operation, and are commonest in those cases where a postoperative evisceration has been repaired in the past. Such hernias usually require operative repair. Although this generally results in a cure, it sometimes takes more than one procedure and may require the introduction of plastic mesh.

SURGICAL SHOCK AND RELATED COMPLICATIONS

- *Surgical Shock*

  This, as we have noted, may occur during operation and postoperatively, and is characterized by a falling blood pressure and cardiovascular collapse. Since its major cause is a reduction in the blood volume, adequate fluid volume replacement becomes of paramount importance, although in some varieties known as *septic shock* the cellular changes caused by infection are the main element in the syndrome.

- *Cardiogenic Shock*

  This is usually due to an acute attack of coronary artery blockage, and requires instantaneous resuscitation measures.

  Unfortunately, over 50 percent of these patients do not survive.

- *Cardiac Arrest* (Heart Stoppage)

  This may occur during the initiation of general anesthesia, during the operation or in the patient's early recovery from the anesthetic. Inadequate oxygen supply and adverse reaction to the anesthetic agent are leading causes. The availability of the emergency "crash cart", the great advances in "CPR" (cardiopulmonary resuscitation) techniques, electrical reversal of abnormal rhythms, and the employment of intravenous drugs and solutions of chemical compounds in conjunction with accurate monitoring of the critical patient, have all contributed to the progressive lowering of mortality in this catastrophe. An unimpeded airway should always be of the utmost importance and the passage of an endotracheal tube can sometimes produce spectacular results in such cases.

ACUTE KIDNEY FAILURE

- Pre-existing Kidney Problems
  This may be due to pre-existing advanced renal disease, or to obstructive conditions in the urinary tract (from kidney to urethra), of which prostatic disease is the commonest.
- Surgical (or *Hypovolemic*) Shock
  The form of kidney failure which is of the greatest importance to the anesthetist and surgeon is that due to a reduction of the heart's output of blood, such as the situation encountered in surgical shock.
- Mismatched Donor's Blood
  Another potent cause of kidney failure is the mismatched blood transfusion, which causes the free hemoglobin released by the reaction to be deposited in the kidney's fine tubules.
- Crush Injuries
  Kidney failure is often seen in severe crush injuries, where *myoglobin*, the muscle's equivalent of hemoglobin, is released and causes kidney blockage. Renal dialysis (by means of an artificial kidney) in such cases may be absolutely lifesaving.
  More importantly, wherever the possibility of kidney failure can be anticipated, essential prophylactic measures can be taken. Intravenous fluids and chemicals that can increase the blood flow through the kidney's filtration system are two such measures.

NEUROLOGICAL COMPLICATIONS (Pertaining to the Nervous System)

- Those following Cardiac Arrest
  These may occur especially if the heart stoppage lasts for more than five minutes, and they may be followed by permanent brain damage or death from deprivation of the brain's oxygen supply. The degree of

damage depends to a great extent on the patient's previous condition and whether the arrest occurred during general anesthesia or after recovery from the anesthetic.

- Massive *Air Embolism*
  This is commonest in cardiac catheterization and in operations on the heart. In this condition air may enter the heart and the arterial circulation to the brain. It may also occur with a major entry of air into an intravenous infusion. The results may be confusion, unconsciousness, various focal paralyses (restricted to a particular set of muscles) or death.
- *Fat Embolism*
  This has been previously mentioned in connection with the lungs, but it may also affect the brain. Fat is released from the bone marrow in major bone fractures or sometimes from operations on major bones, and droplets of fat which are released into the blood stream may reach the brain and produce symptoms of neurological impairment, commencing with confusion.
- Strokes
  These may occur when an undue rise in blood pressure causes the rupture of a weakened blood vessel in the brain, or when an undue drop in the blood pressure causes a blood clot to form in a diseased and narrowed artery in the brain.
- Injuries to the Spinal Cord
  These may occur where the blood supply to a particular level of the spinal cord is cut off during the course of an operation such as the repair of an *abdominal aortic aneurysm,* a condition in which the major arterial trunk in the abdomen is dangerously ballooned. They may also occur as the severest complication of spinal anesthesia.
- Injuries to the Peripheral Nerves
  These may be due to inadvertent damage during an operation, but cases where the injury results from incorrect positioning of the patient are also far from uncommon. In such cases the damage may be the result of prolonged pressure or undue traction on the peripheral nerves in the unconscious individual. Lesser degrees of injury may occur due to careless deep injections.
- Persistent Pain in the Operative Scar
  This may be due to tiny nerve fibres getting caught in the scar tissue or the actual formation of a neuroma in the scar: a neuroma is a tender and painful bulbous swelling on the cut end of a nerve, and may have to be excised to relieve the symptoms.

NUTRITIONAL PROBLEMS

All the known complications of operative surgery, including those of the associated anesthesia, are magnified by inadequate nutrition. The requirements of adequate essential proteins, fats, and carbohydrates are of the utmost importance in the operative and postoperative patient. So are the vitamin, fluid and *electrolyte* requirements. These electrolytes include sodium, potassium, calcium, magnesium, and chlorides, iron, bicarbonate, and the so-called trace metals, such as zinc and cobalt.

Methods of artificial maintenance of nutrition are necessary in those cases where the patient is unable to ingest the required amount by mouth, where there is obstruction in the digestive tract—mechanical or neurological—or where there is failure of absorption or utilization. These methods include intravenous infusions, either via a peripheral limb vein or a major "central" vein; a feeding-tube into the stomach, via the nose or mouth, or a feeding *gastrostomy* or *jejunostomy*.

In a gastrostomy, a small abdominal incision exposes the front of the stomach, which is perforated to introduce a catheter in a valvular fashion to prevent leakage. The catheter is tethered to the stomach, then brought out to the skin away from the incision, and securely anchored to the skin puncture site. This tube can be used for high-calorie, high-vitamin feeding, and for intermittent decompression of the stomach.

In a jejunostomy, a similar procedure is carried out, using the upper portion of the small intestine, and with an appropriate valvular technique, but intermittent decompression is not required. The advantage of the jejunostomy is that there are no problems with delayed outflow from the stomach or with the consequent regurgitation and possible aspiration into the respiratory passages.

Complications

- Leakage
  Occasionally the catheter of a gastrostomy or jejunostomy may be inadvertently pulled out. It should be replaced immediately with the utmost care and with maximum lighting, otherwise the catheter may be lodged outside the stomach or jejunum. This will result in the solu-

tion of nutrients leaking into the abdominal cavity and leading to the development of peritonitis.

Intravenous nutritional support is used when there is no possibility of getting an adequate level of nutrition via the digestive tract, otherwise the tube "ostomies" just described may be employed to advantage. In either case the essential proteins are actually given in a more simplified chemical form, namely, the amino acids that are the small component parts of all proteins.

Complications

- Inflammation
  In peripheral vein infusions (such as an IV in the upper limb) the vein may become acutely inflamed and/or blocked, or even seriously infected (acute *thrombophlebitis*).
- Infection
  An indwelling central venous catheter may become infected, with septic bloodstream spread and, especially, bloodborne invasion by *candida albicans*, a variety of yeast.
- Ulceration
  Occasionally the catheter may ulcerate through the vein wall, causing internal bleeding or leakage of the fluid into the chest cavity (the *pleural cavity*).
- Infected Blood Clots
  In the event of an infected bloodclot breaking loose from the infected vein it may set up abscesses in distant locations.
  This complication is known as *septic embolism*.

CHAPTER 4

Appendectomy and Hernia Repairs

Removal of a normal appendix or a mildly inflamed appendix is one of the most straightforward operations and carries no particular risks, other than the overall risks of all surgery and anesthesia. On the other hand, a severely infected appendix, one that has developed into a pus-bag or has become gangrenous, and especially one that has ruptured, can be extremely dangerous and fraught with complications. These include acute generalized peritonitis, intraabdominal abscesses and septicemia.

The appendix may be tied down deep in the pelvis by *adhesions* (the abnormal sticking together of tissues or anatomical structures), or be located high up behind the liver, and may be very hard to get at through the usual small incision.

Complications

- Abscesses
  Abscess formation may occur in the pelvis, where it is easiest to diagnose and to drain, or below the diaphragm, where it is hardest to diagnose and to drain.
- Wound Infection
  There are two forms of wound infection that deserve separate mention. The first is known as *crepitant cellulitis*, a solid inflammation with gas bubbles in the soft tissues. This may be caused by the bacteria of gas gangrene, but is sometimes due to other anaerobic bacteria (that thrive in the absence of oxygen). The second is known as

symbiotic gangrene, in which two different types of bacteria combine forces to produce death of skin and soft tissues.
- Scarring
Appendectomy wounds that require drainage are prone to develop ugly depressed scars, and are a source of potential weakness with the subsequent development of *incisional hernia*.
- Leakage
Occasionally the stump of the appendix may be inadequately secured, with resultant leakage into the abdominal cavity and either generalized peritonitis or abscess formation.
- Inversion Problem
The inverted stump may telescope itself further into the adjoining large bowel, producing what is known as an *intussusception*.
- Bleeding
On rare occasions bleeding may occur into the bowel from a small blood vessel in the stump of the appendix.
- Fistula
Sometimes it turns out that the appendix is involved in an intestinal inflammation known as *Crohn's disease*. In these cases, following appendectomy, a *fistula* may develop, that is an infected tract extending from the stump of the appendix to the skin and discharging pus or fecal fluid.
- Multiple Liver Abscesses
These may occur in a complication named *pylephlebitis*, a condition where blood clots in the veins that drain the appendix become infected and the septic clot reaches the liver.
- Lung Abscesses
These may occur if septic clots form in the main systemic veins—as in the pelvis—and travel to the lung circulation.
- Putrid Brain Abscesses
These may occur if septic clots reach the arterial side of the circulation and pass into the *carotid* artery to the brain.
In all three such varieties of septic clots there is usually an accompanying septicemia.
- Early Postoperative Adhesions
These may develop in the first week or two and produce early postoperative bowel obstruction.
- Late Postoperative Adhesions
As a late complication of appendectomy, these are usually quite harmless and do not produce symptoms except when they happen to

cause intestinal obstruction—by kinking or constriction due to a tight band.

Most symptoms attributed to adhesions are misdiagnosed. Such symptoms may represent simple indigestion or a more serious abdominal disorder requiring investigation. It should be realized that adhesions are usually a result of a healing process in which the mechanisms to limit the spread of infection in an area result in a fibrous connection between organs or tissue layers.

HERNIA REPAIRS

All hernias, commonly known as "ruptures", have certain common features. They consist of a *hernial sac*, a protrusion of the silk-like lining of the abdominal cavity (known as the *peritoneum*), through an aperture in the muscle layers—either congenital or acquired—and containing intestine or other abdominal contents, or often just fluid or no contents at all. The operation, therefore, consists of the removal of the peritoneal sac, restoring the contents to the abdomen, and a repair of the muscular defect.

Classification

Inguinal hernia: located just above the groin.

Scrotal hernia: an inguinal hernia which has progressed downwards into the scrotal sac.

Femoral hernia: located just below the groin, in the uppermost thigh.

Umbilical hernia: located at the navel.

Epigastric hernia: located in the upper abdomen.

Ventral hernia: an abdominal hernia other than the above and associated with a separation or weakening of abdominal muscles.

Incisional hernia: occurs at the site of any previous abdominal wound, especially one that was disrupted (opened up—as in "burst abdomen").

Diaphragmatic hernia: may be congenital, which usually requires early repair. The congenital type is usually associated with the presence of a major portion of the gastrointestinal tract in the chest and with compression of the lung.

The adult type is usually a widening of the opening for the *esophagus* (the gullet) to pass from the chest into the abdomen. Since this opening is called the *esophageal hiatus*, this type of hernia is called a *hiatus hernia*. (see P.52)

Hernias may be reducible: disappearing on lying down or with gentle pressure, or irreducible: failing to disappear. They may be accompanied by obstruction of a loop of bowel which is trapped in the hernial sac, or by what is called *strangulation* of the intestine, a term which means that the trapped bowel has its blood supply shut off by the entrapment. Such strangulated bowel may proceed to local gangrene, perforation, and peritonitis.

Complications

- Recurrence of the Hernia
  The most important complication of hernial repair is recurrence, which may be early or late. Operative factors are failure to remove the hernial sac completely, poor suturing techniques, and the use of absorbable rather than nonabsorbable sutures. Patient factors are obesity, poor tissues which are unable to retain the sutures and really require the surgical use of plastic patches, severe postoperative distension, diabetes, malnutrition, and lung disease with excessive coughing.
- Injury to Adjacent Structures
  There are several structures which may be inadvertently injured during hernial repair are several. They include severing of the *vas deferens*, (the duct which carries semen from the testicle) and damage to the blood supply of the testicle in the male, or to the sensory nerve of the groin area, with pain and numbness in that region. On rare occasions the urinary bladder may be injured, as may a trapped loop of bowel in a constriction ring that has to be released. Injury to the colon is more likely to occur in a variety of inguinal hernia known as a *sliding hernia*, in which the colon and its blood supply are outside the hernial sac but form part of its peritoneal lining.

- *Hematoma* (A Collection of Blood in the Tissues)
  Persistent bleeding fom any small bloodvessel that has been inadequately secured may produce a hematoma in the wound, either fluid or clotted, and requiring drainage.
- *Seroma* (A Collection of Serum in the Wound)
  This can be readily evacuated by needle and syringe.
- Infection
  Wound infection following hernial repairs may occur in the circumstances that are common to all surgical procedures, but will obviously be more common with strangulated hernias or where there has been an injury to the bowel. It will also be more common in those cases that require the use of plastic mesh, or large sutures of multifilament nonabsorbable material (because bacteria can easily lodge and persist in such foreign, nonbiological material).
- Scrotal Swelling
  Scrotal *hydrocele* is a condition in which clear fluid collects in the scrotal sac, and may occur if part of the hernial sac is left in the scrotum. There may also be swelling of the scrotal skin or of the testicle from compression of the veins in the *spermatic cord* (the cord leading to the testicle), or from a repair which is too tight. This particular group of swelling complications usually resolves in time.
- Abnormal Clotting
  Rarely, in the repair of a femoral hernia, the main vein of the lower limb may be compressed, and *thrombosis* may follow, causing obstruction of the bloodflow by clot in the vein, or—at the worst—the spread of blood clots in the bloodstream, known as *embolism*.

CHAPTER 5

Operations on the Esophagus

These include operations for cancer, for noncancerous obstructive conditions, and for *reflux esophagitis*, caused by regurgitation of acid or alkaline contents from the stomach into the gullet—with or without associated repair of a diaphragmatic hernia. The *esophagus* is the medical name for the gullet which carries food from the throat cavity to the stomach. The *diaphragm* is the muscular sheet which separates the contents of the chest (heart and lungs, etc) from those of the abdomen (the stomach and intestines, etc). The esophagus extends downwards in the chest, behind the heart and lungs, and goes through an opening in the diaphragm to join the stomach at its upper end, known as the *cardia*.

SURGERY FOR CANCER OF THE ESOPHAGUS

This operation consists of removing the entire esophagus and adjoining upper end of the stomach, then freeing up the stomach as completely as possible while still maintaining its bloodsupply. Finally the mobilized stomach is brought up through the chest and joined to the upper cut end of the esophagus in the lower neck. If this proves impossible then the colon (specially cleansed prior to operation) is used as an isolated segment—with its intact bloodvessels—and joined to the stomach below and to the cut end of the esophagus above, in the lower neck. Sometimes a segment of the upper small intestine (*jejunum*) is used instead. For cancers at the junction of the stomach and esophagus the upper half of the stomach and lower third of the esophagus are removed, and the remaining stomach is mobilized into the chest cavity where it is joined to the cut end of the esophagus.

Complications

- Leakage and Infection
  Leakage can occur at the point or points where the joins are made (*anastomoses*), either with sutures or with staples. This may lead to a draining *fistula* in the lower neck, infection of the chest space (*pleural space*)—a condition known as *empyema*—or infection of the soft tissue space between the pleural cavities—a condition known as *mediastinitis*. If the leakage is below the diaphragm, peritonitis may ensue, either generalized, or forming an abscess below the diaphragm (*subphrenic abscess*).
- Blockage of the Arterial Blood Supply
  This can occur due to kinking or stretching of the vessels, or actual interruption of the blood supply during a difficult mobilisation of either the stomach, jejunum, or the interposed colonic segment. It will result in the death of the affected tissue, segment or organ.
- *Esophageal Reflux* (Regurgitation)
  This may be due to a failure to provide a valvular anastomosis between the stomach or intestinal segment and the cut end of the esophagus. It may lead to aspiration pneumonia.
- Obstruction
  Mechanical obstruction may occur at any of the anastomoses due to local scarring and resulting constriction. Neurological obstruction may occur at the outlet of the stomach, due to division of the vagus nerves to the stomach in the course of resecting the esophagus, and can be avoided by dividing a ring of muscle at the outlet of the stomach, called the *pylorus*.

OPERATIONS FOR NONCANCEROUS CONDITIONS OF THE ESOPHAGUS

Achalasia of the Cardia

This is a condition in which the swallowing mechanism at the lower end of the esophagus is disturbed and the muscle ring at the entrance to the stomach fails to relax. The esophagus becomes grossly dilated due to obstruction and the patient becomes progressively starved. Aside from instrumental dilatation, the commonest treatment is an operation called the *Heller procedure*, in which the malfunctioning ring of muscle is divided.

Complications

- Failure to Cure the Condition
  This includes failure due to inadequate division of the muscle or perforation because the incision was too deep. If the incision in the muscle is too long, the patient may experience postoperative esophageal regurgitation.
- Diaphragmatic Hernia
  This may result from failure to repair the widened opening in the diaphragm adequately.

Reflux Esophagitis

This condition can occur with or without diaphragmatic hernia. It occurs when medical treatment fails to control the regurgitation of acid gastric contents (or, sometimes, alkaline upper intestinal contents) into the lower esophagus. The operation is generally a wrap-around procedure to produce an antireflux valve at the entrance to the stomach. A repair of the associated hernia, when present, is performed at the same time. The hernia in such cases—known as a *hiatus hernia*—is a widening of the muscular aperture through which the esophagus passes from the thorax into the abdomen, permitting the upper portion of the stomach to migrate into the lower thorax.

Complications

- Recurrence of Reflux Symptoms
  This is due to failure to produce a functional valve at the entrance of the esophagus into the stomach. It may also be due to slipping of the wrap-around from its original position.
- Too Tight a Repair
  This may produce obstructive symptoms such as difficulty in swallowing, or gas bloating and inability to belch.
- Injury to the Spleen
  In the past, this usually led to removal of the spleen. In recent years there has been a much greater effort to repair and preserve the spleen.
- Development of a new Hiatus Hernia
  This hernia, in which the fundus of the stomach slips into the chest alongside the esophagus, is a late complication.

CHAPTER 6

Operations on the Stomach and Small Intestine

Gastric and Duodenal Ulcers

Operations for gastric or duodenal ulcer are much less frequent than they were just a few decades ago, because of improved medical management of the problem. They are also far less radical, although there are some surgeons who still prefer the older procedures and can demonstrate excellent results. Previously, the operation consisted of removing a major part of the stomach and joining up the gastric stump either directly to the *duodenum* (the very first part of the small intestine) or closing the cut end of the duodenum and anastomosing the stomach to the side of the upper small intestine known as the *jejunum*.

VAGOTOMY AND PYLOROPLASTY OR DISTAL GASTRECTOMY

As noted above, the operation formerly performed for gastric or duodenal ulcer that failed to be controlled with medical treatment, was partial removal (up to four fifths) of the stomach and, when properly performed, gave good results. The newer operative approach, which is really reserved for the complications of the ulcer and for failure of medical treatment, is directed towards reducing the gastric acidity and establishing an adequate outlet for the gastric contents. This is done by removing segments of the *vagus nerves*, which control the acid secretion and the motility of the stomach, and either modifying the outlet (called a *pyloroplasty*) or creating a new outlet. Some surgeons prefer to remove the terminal portion of the stomach along with the vagotomy (called *distal gastrectomy*).

GASTRECTOMY (Removal of the Stomach)

This can be either partial, total, or with a portion of the esophagus, and with either type of outlet revision. The direct joining (anastomosis) to the duodenum is known as the *Billroth 1* procedure and the indirect anastomosis, to the jejunum, is known as the *Billroth 2* procedure, in memory of the great turn-of-the century German surgeon, Theodore Billroth.

Complications of Gastric Surgery

- Persistent Bleeding
  Following surgery, this may be due to bleeding from the anastomosis or the pyloroplasty. It may be from an ulcer that has been left behind. If the operation is done for bleeding ulcer as an emergency procedure, it is customary to oversew the bleeding vessel in the ulcer bed, making sure that the bleeding is arrested on tying the suture. Of course, persistent bleeding may be due to an uncorrected clotting defect. Bleeding may occur outside the stomach or intestinal interior by virtue of one of the feeder vessels, especially an artery, that continues to bleed if it has not been tied or a clip applied at surgery, or if either of these have loosened.
- Leakage
  This may occur at the pyloroplasty or anastomosis and may result in a duodenal fistula, with external drainage of gastrointestinal juices.
- Generalized Peritonitis
  This is the worst result of leakage.
- Subphrenic Abscess
  An abscess under the diaphragm may result from leakage.
- Obstruction
  This may occur at the pyloroplasty or the anastomosis. It may result from entrapment of an intestinal loop through an aperture, or due to severe kinking. Obstruction may also be the result of adhesions, either early or late.
- Postoperative *Acute Pancreatitis*
  This is a rapidly developing inflammation of the pancreas, and may occur as a result of injury to that organ in the course of operations on the stomach and duodenum. It is extremely serious and carries a high mortality.

- Rupture of the Esophagus
  This is a rare and extremely grave occurrence with vagotomy, and is more likely if there has been previous surgery in this region.
- Injury To The Spleen
  This is much less common than with operations at the lower end of the esophagus. Here, again, the modern surgical trend is to try and repair and preserve the organ rather than removing it routinely when damaged.
- *Postoperative Jaundice*
  Yellow discolouration of the eyes and skin may be due to actual injury to the common bile duct during a gastrectomy. It may also be due to inflammatory swelling around the duodenum, with temporary bile duct obstruction, bile spillage at operation, duodenal leakage, or break-up of red blood corpuscles in the bloodstream.
- Gastric Retention
  The hold-up of stomach contents following stomach surgery may be due to an unsatisfactory emptying mechanism, with the danger of regurgitation and aspiration. Aside from a true obstruction requiring surgical relief, the commonest cause is temporary swelling at the anastomosis. It may also occur as a temporary side effect of vagotomy (since division of the vagus nerves slows down emptying), but, if the muscular ring—known as the *pyloric sphincter*—controlling the normal gastric outlet, is not adequately divided at the time of vagotomy, the gastric retention may persist.
- Recurrent Ulceration
  Following gastrectomy of the Billroth 2 variety, recurrent ulceration may occur just beyond the junction between the gastric stump and the jejunum, with intractable pain, bleeding or even perforation. *Gastro-jejuno-colic fistula* is a dreaded complication which may follow extension of such recurrent ulceration to form a communication between the anastomosis and a segment of colon adherent to the penetrating ulcer.
- The *Dumping Syndrome*
  This is a complication of almost any of the aforementioned gastric operations. It is least common in vagotomy and pyloroplasty. The symptoms come on after meals and include the following; upper abdominal discomfort, nausea, weakness, belching, sweating, rapid pulse, hot flushes, and sometimes vomiting or diarrhea.
- *Alkaline Reflux Gastritis or Esophagitis*
  This is a condition in which the alkaline contents of the small intestine enter the stomach interior after gastric surgery and sets up an

inflammation; if these contents are regurgitated into the lower esophagus, the inflammation may be at least as severe as the more common acid reflux esophagitis. It should be mentioned that *hiatus hernia*—the usual kind of diaphragmatic hernia—may result from vagotomy or high gastric resections and contribute to esophageal reflux.
- Chronic Diarrhea
This is one of several unpleasant forms of postoperative digestive upset. Another is failure of appetite and chronic weight loss.
- Absorption Defects
There may be disturbed absorption of vitamins and minerals, especially iron and calcium. Iron metabolism may be disturbed following gastrectomy and cause chronic anemia.
- Gallstones
There appears to be an increased tendency to develop this condition after vagotomy and pyloroplasty.

RADICAL GASTRECTOMY FOR STOMACH CANCER

This is usually far more extensive than that for gastric or duodenal ulcer. Accordingly, the risks of postoperative complications are far greater then those mentioned above for gastrectomy. Since they are essentially the same as those previously listed, they need no further elaboration. Of special significance in this respect is the degree to which neighbouring structures are involved and may be included in the resection. The spleen, which may easily be injured during high gastric surgery (or low esophageal and hiatus surgery) is often removed in cancer gastrectomies rather than repaired and preserved.

OPERATIONS ON THE SMALL INTESTINE

Small bowel obstruction

This is the commonest reason for operating on the small intestine. The causes of such obstruction include the following conditions:

Postoperative adhesions, following previous abdominal or pelvic surgery.

Volvulus, or twisting of the bowel.

38   Informed Consent to Surgery

"Foreign bodies", or undigested food lodged in the intestine.

Tumours in the intestine, surrounding or compressing it.

Obstruction of a loop of bowel in a hernia.

Obstruction in association with strangulation (an interruption of the blood supply), as in thrombosis or embolism involving the intestines blood vessels, or strangulated hernia (see Chapter 4).

Intussusception, a condition in which the intestine telescopes itself by turning into the next portion, usually progressing itself forwards, towards or through the colon.

OPERATIONS FOR SMALL BOWEL OBSTRUCTION

Small bowel obstruction is the commonest reason for operating on the small intestine, and the commonest cause of such obstruction is postoperative adhesions following previous abdominal or pelvic surgery. Conversely, it is doubtful whether adhesions cause symptoms in the absence of obstruction.

As a basic rule, an acute onset of obstruction is essentially a sign of small bowel involvement while a slow development of obstruction is typical of large bowel involvement, although in the final stage it, too, may become an acute emergency.

The symptoms of small intestine obstruction are intermittent colicky abdominal pains, vomiting, inability to pass rectal gas, and distension of the entire belly.

The actual operations include separation of adhesions, which may lead to tears in the bowel-wall, resections of badly damaged bowel or areas of damaged blood supply, and suction decompression of grossly distended bowel with a special tube inserted through a small opening in the bowel.

Complications

- Regurgitation and Aspiration
  Prior to administering the anesthetic, it is important to be aware of

the possibility of regurgitation of intestinal contents and aspiration of highly toxic and infected fluid into the lungs.
- Leakage
The greatest danger during an operation for obstruction of the small intestine is contamination of the abdominal cavity with leaking intestinal fluid. This may lead to generalized peritonitis or intraabdominal abscesses, to a far more dangerous degree than would occur from leakage in the absence of obstruction.
- Fistula
When an abscess that involves small bowel discharges to the exterior, or when a loop of small intestine is adherent to the abdominal wall and is perforated, a fistula may result, with massive outpouring of intestinal fluid through an opening in the skin. Such a fistula may be associated with dramatic nutritional loss to the patient, and is a very difficult complication to manage.
- Fluid and Electrolyte Problems
Another secondary complication of small intestinal fistula is disturbance of fluid and electrolyte balance. (*Electrolytes* are inorganic constituents such as sodium, potassium, and chlorides). Protein loss may affect the balance between the fluids in the blood stream and those in the soft tissue spaces; this can produce accumulation of fluids in the soft tissues, with swelling of the lower limbs and lower trunk, especially the lower back in the bedridden patient.
- Nutritional Deficiency of Mechanical Origin
Small bowel deficit is a complication resulting from a major resection of small intestine in such conditions as *Crohn's Disease*, an inflammatory rather than infective bowel disease. The extreme shortening of available digestive lining results in severe nutritional deficiency.
- Escape of Small Bowel through the Wound
Abdominal dehiscence with evisceration (in which the wound opens up and the intestines protrude) is a major danger of any operation on the small intestine. Gross distension and wound contamination are major factors. Others are a persistent, ineffectual cough, or unrelieved retching.

CHAPTER 7

Operations on the Colon, Rectum and Anus

COLON RESECTIONS

The leading indication for colonic surgery is cancer.

A cancer of the right colon (*ascending colon* plus *cecum*) is treated by removal of the right half of the colon and *anastomosing* (joining up two structures, usually of the hollow variety) the terminal small bowel to the cut end of the colon.

Cancer of the intermediate section of large bowel (*transverse colon*) is dealt with by removing that portion of the colon with disease-free margins and joining the cut ends.

Cancer of the left colon (*descending colon*) is treated by removal of the left half of the colon and end-to-end anastomosis.

Cancer of the *sigmoid colon* (the large segment in the pelvis) is treated by removal of that segment with cancer-free margins and anastomosis to the rectum. It should be mentioned at this point that in recent years more and more anastomoses in the digestive tract are being done with stapling machines rather than with sutures.

Complications of colon surgery

- Spillage of Colonic Contents
  Those complications related to such spillage are frequent, often multiple, and often preventable. Preparation of the bowel interior is most important and includes mechanical emptying and cleansing, the ad-

ministration of antibacterial agents, and in some instances antifungal agents. The reason for these precautions is the fact that spillage of colonic contents is far more lethal than spillage of small intestinal contents during surgery. Of course, obstruction, perforation or abscess formation makes this hazard far greater.

Complications of right colon resection

- Injury to the Duodenum
- Injury to the Major Intestinal Blood Vessels
  (in the upper right and central abdomen).
- Failure of the Anastomosis
  This is between the small and large intestine and may occur due to impairment of the blood supply, or to technical defects, resulting in leakage and fistula.

Complications of transverse colon resections

- These are similar to those of transverse colectomy, but are mostly due to inadequate mobilization of the two sides of the colon prior to joining up the cut ends, thus placing too much tension on the anastomotic suture line and producing leakage.

Complications of left colon resections

- Injury to the Spleen.
- Injury to the *Ureter* (the Tube from the Kidney to the Bladder)
- Bleeding from the Colonic Bed
  This occurs in the soft tissue gutter from which the left colon was removed.

These operative injuries are particularly prone to occur in resections for a common condition known as *diverticulitis*. This is a disease in which small pouches occur—like tiny hernias—in the wall of the colon, and set up an inflammation that may eventually require surgery.

Complications of *sigmoid colon* resections

This means removal of the terminal portion of the colon.
If the anastomosis is to the lower rectum—as for cancer—then it is known as an *anterior resection* (see below).

- The complications of resecting the sigmoid colon include the aforementioned, but are often particularly due to inadequate mobilization of the left colon prior to resection. Another factor is failure to ensure an adequate blood supply to the anastomotic area.

Complications of total colectomy

This operation, removal of the entire colon, is usually performed for advanced inflammatory disease of the colon, especially that form known as *ulcerative colitis*. It is also performed in cases of multiple *polyps* (small berrylike tumours, usually benign but sometimes premalignant) which can affect the entire colon.

- The complications of total colectomy combine all those mentioned under segmental colectomy plus those due to the disease itself and its preoperative treatment with steroids (cortisones). The patients are often debilitated and have extremely poor healing powers, which are made worse by the steroids. There is also an increased danger of postoperative shock and postoperative bleeding.
- Recurrent Disease
  When the rectum is retained there may be a recurrence of severe ulcerative colitis in the rectal remnant that will require secondary surgery.

Abdominoperineal Resection
This operation consists of removing the rectum along with all or part of the colon (see below).

COLOSTOMY

This is an opening in the colon which is joined to the skin and through which the colon can evacuate its contents into a special bag-appliance. It may be temporary or permanent.

As a temporary device, its main use is as a first stage in colonic surgery where there is an element of obstruction, and it may be closed after the definitive surgery has been completed successfully. It may also be used to supplement a one-stage colonic resection where the colon is not empty at the time of surgery. A permanent colostomy is used in those operations in which the rectum has been removed.

Complications

The recorded incidence of complications in colostomy is surprisingly high but can be considerably diminished by a simple observance of careful operative techniques.
The formidable list includes the following:
- Hernia Around the Opening
- Stricture at the Outlet
- Prolapse (Gross Protrusion)
- Retraction
- Obstruction
- Perforation
- Fistulous Tracts
- Abscess (and Miscellaneous other Complications).

TUBE CECOSTOMY

This is a temporary drainage of the first part of the large bowel and can be used to supplement a resection of the left colon as a blow-off valve to protect the distal anastomosis, but should not be used in the presence of obstruction.

Complications

- Although an assortment of complications has been reported, the performance of a temporary tube cecostomy, properly managed, should have almost no complications relative to the procedure and the opening should close spontaneously following removal. Of course, if cecostomy is erroneously employed in the presence of colonic obstruction, or other than as a blow- off device to protect a leftsided colon resection, then the complication rate will be high.
- Cecostomy performed in the presence of cecal disease, local abscess, or the debilitated patient, may require secondary surgery to effect closure or bypass.

ILEOSTOMY

This operation is done when a total colectomy is performed.
It consists of opening the terminal small intestine onto the skin of the lower right abdomen. The ileostomy empties into a special watertight

collecting device worn by the patient, or an *ileal pouch* is constructed by the surgeon. Such pouches are fashioned from the terminal small bowel and may be located just underneath the ileostomy outlet as a receptacle for liquid feces which can be emptied periodically by a tube inserted by the patient. (A similar pouch may be constructed as a substitute for the rectum when the small intestine is joined to the anus).

Complications

- Obstruction
- Leakage
- Inflammation
- Perforation
- Hernia Around the Ileostomy Opening
- Fistulous Tracts
- Persistent Malfunction

In multiple polyposis requiring total colectomy the small intestine is sutured to the rectum without ileostomy and the complications are far less than with ulcerative colitis.

OPERATIONS ON THE RECTUM AND ANUS

ANTERIOR RESECTION (of the Sigmoid Colon and Upper Rectum)

This may be complicated by the factors previously outlined under Colon Resections, but they have been considerably reduced by the employment of stapling devices for the difficult anastomosis at a low level.

Complications

- Persistent Pelvic Bleeding
- Collection of a large Pelvic Hematoma
- Failure of the Anastomosis
  This may be due to deficient blood supply to the anastomosis and lead to leakage.
- Stricture Formation at the Anastomosis
- Fistula

ABDOMINOPERINEAL RESECTION

In this operation, the rectum and anal canal are completely removed, and the complications of anastomosis are thereby avoided. A permanent colostomy is an essential part of the operation.

Complications

- Bleeding
  Persistent pelvic bleeding is the most common and serious complication. The chances of troublesome pelvic bleeding are greater than with the other segmental resections.
- Impotence
  In the younger male, a difficult pelvic dissection may damage the nerves controlling the patient's sexual functions.
- Small Bowel Obstruction
  This may occur in the pelvis, due to abscess formation or adhesions.
- Obstructed or Strangulated Intestine
  A trapped loop of small intestine at the bottom of the pelvis may be undetected and if it becomes obstructed or—even worse—strangulated, the results may be fatal.
- Urinary Problems
  Bladder infection and urinary obstruction are more common in male patients, particularly in elderly men.
- Injury to Adjacent Structures
  Operative injuries to the ureters, bladder, and urethra, may occur during the operative dissection, and should be repaired—if possible during the operation.
- Problems with the Perineal Scar
  Persistent pain and *sinus* formation (a discharging tract to the skin, but one which does not communicate with a hollow organ) in the perineal scar. This usually means the presence of residual or recurrent cancer, where the operation has been performed for malignancy.
- Abscesses
  Where the operation has been performed for chronic inflammatory bowel disease (Ulcerative Colitis or Crohn's Disease) there may be late abscesses and sinus formation in the perineal scar, which can become quite deep and extensive.

These complications are mostly preventable and treatable by correct measures.

46 Informed Consent to Surgery

HEMORRHOIDECTOMY (Removal of Anal Piles)

Complications

- Persistent urinary retention
- Persistent bleeding
- Persistent inability to evacuate stool
- Delayed stricture of the anal ring, due to scarring

These complications are largely preventable and frequently overstated, as is the fear of unmanageable pain, and the operation deserves a much better reputation if correctly performed and managed.

SURGERY FOR ANAL FISTULA AND PILONIDAL SINUS

Anal fistula is a condition in which there is a channel between the interior of the anal canal and the surrounding skin, with discharge of pus and fecal material.

- **The Commonest Complication** of operations to cure anal fistula is recurrence, and the same is true of operations for *Pilonidal Sinus* (one or more discharging sinuses in the tail-bone region, usually containing impacted tufts of hair, and periodically producing abscesses).

SURGERY FOR *ANAL FISSURE*

This condition is a painful crack in the anal skin, associated with pain and spasm.

- **The Main Complication** is recurrence following a misguided attempt to excise the fissure itself, rather than releving the muscle spasm by nonoperative methods and, if these fail, by dividing a few muscle fibres at the appropriate level to break the cycle of spasm. This operation is known as *internal sphincterotomy*.

CHAPTER 8

Operations on the Digestive Tract of Infants

Most operations on the digestive tract of infants are done for a wide variety of congenital defects. The initial part of these operations consists of *laparotomy* (opening the belly).

When the abdomen is being explored for congenital abnormalities, obstructions, or perforations in the newborn, an adequate incision is vital, in order to visualize the whole of the small intestine and most of the colon and exclude unsuspected additional defects. When the exact location of the condition to be dealt with is known, the incision may be placed precisely.

The most common of these is the condition *called congenital hypertrophic pyloric stenosis.* It is caused by a highly overdeveloped muscular ring (*the pyloric sphincter*) at the outlet of the stomach, resulting in total gastric obstruction.

THE *RAMSTEDT PROCEDURE*

This is the name of the operation to cure this condition. Its main feature is a complete division of the pyloric sphincter and it has a very high success rate.

Complications

- Aspiration of Gastric Contents into the Air Passages
- Dehydration and Electrolyte Disturbance

- Perforation of the Duodenum
  This may occur during the operation, with leakage of bile. (It should be understood that newborn infantile tissues are extremely fragile and prone to operative injury).
- Operative Hemorrhage
  This is most unusual.
- Postoperative Vomiting
  This usually clears up spontaneously.
- Disruption of the Wound and Evisceration
  This requires secondary repair.

SURGERY FOR DUODENAL OBSTRUCTION AND ABNORMALITIES

These are congenital conditions affecting the first loop of small intestine into which the stomach normally empties its contents. In most cases the operation is essentially an appropriate bypass procedure.

Complications

- Leakage
- Peritonitis
- Delayed Function
  This is usually self-limiting
- Undetected additional congenital defects

SURGERY FOR JEJUNAL AND ILEAL OBSTRUCTIONS AND ABNORMALITIES

These are congenital conditions affecting the second and third parts of the small intestine. Some of these can involve extremely difficult surgery, including segmental resections and awkward anastomoses.

Complications

- These operations may be followed by the same complications as those described for the general population, but at a much higher risk. Delayed return of function and undetected congenital defects are additional complications.

SURGERY FOR *MECONIUM ILEUS*

In this condition the intestinal contents of the newborn, known as *meconium*, in contrast to feces, is too viscous to permit normal emptying and produces a glue-like obstruction of the small bowel.

Complications

- The association of the defect with cystic fibrosis makes the possibility of respiratory complications very much higher.

SURGERY FOR *MECKEL'S DIVERTICULUM*

This is a pouchlike congenital structure, like an additional appendix, located in the terminal loop of small bowel. It occurs in 2 percent of the population. When it becomes acutely inflamed, ulcerated or perforated, the cause of bowel obstruction or intestinal bleeding, its removal may become necessary.

Complications

- These are essentially the same as those of appendectomy.

SURGERY FOR MISCELLANEOUS SMALL BOWEL MALFORMATIONS

These may be in the form of webs in the bowel interior, malrotation (failure of the intestine to reach the normal position at birth), and bowel duplications (double segements of intestine.

Complications

- These are the same as those related to any operations on the small intestine, but with a higher degree of severity in the infant.

SURGERY FOR *HIRSCHSPUNG'S DISEASE*

This condition is a congenital defect in the nerve control of the colon in a segment of that organ, producing infantile bowel obstruction or chronic and severe constipation later on. There may also be attacks of bowel inflammation.

Surgery for this condition includes colostomy and bringing the normal colon (with intact nerve supply) down to the anal ring, to which it is sutured.

Complications

- Sepsis
  The main complications are those of a separated suture line due to excessive tension or inadequate blood supply; this produces fecal contamination, sepsis, retraction of the bowel up into the pelvis and abdomen). Death from overwhelming infection in such cases can only be averted by prompt diverting colostomy and antibacterial therapy.
- Ureteric Injury
  During the operative dissection there is a danger of injury to the ureters.
- Anal Stricture
  A later complication is the development of stricture at the anus.
- Recurrence
  If part of the denervated colon (absence of the essential nerve cells) is left in the sutured colon, there will be a recurrence of Hirschsprung symptoms.

SURGERY FOR *IMPERFORATE ANUS*

This is a condition in which there is congenital absence of the normal anal aperture, which—in the more severe cases—is associated with abnormal internal communications such as to the bladder, urethra or vagina. In such severe cases the surgery consists of a preliminary colostomy followed by a complex repair of the various abnormalities.

Complications

- Anal stenosis
  The commonest postoperative complication is anal narrowing to the point of obstruction, requiring secondary surgery.
- Incontinence
  A more troublesome complication is that of persistent fecal incontinence due to injury or failure to improve the function of the muscles controlling fecal continence at the anal level.

- Urinary problems
  Various urinary abnormalities may be associated with high levels of imperforate anus and, of course, urinary infection is a troublesome secondary problem in all such cases.

CHAPTER 9

Operations on the Biliary System, the Pancreas and Spleen

The commonest of these operations is removal of the gallbladder, *cholecystectomy*, usually for stones. The next commonest is exploration of the bile ducts. These, and related operations, are among the commonest of abdominal operations but may decline with the advent of shock wave fragmentation of stones—without surgery—and the administration of biological solvents in the earliest phase of gallstone formation. A third type of biliary operation is reconstructive surgery of the bile ducts as a result of injury to the bile ducts.

To understand these, it is important to visualize the anatomy of the area. Bile is formed in the liver and collected into the right and left *hepatic ducts* which drain the right and left lobes of the liver. These combine to form the *common bile duct* which proceeds below the liver to traverse the back of the *pancreas* and empties into the duodenum.

Part way down the common bile duct the narrow *cystic duct* connects to the gallbladder, which is attached to the undersurface of the liver. The gallbladder serves to concentrate the bile, so that it can be stored for release through the cystic duct into the common duct whenever fats enter the duodenum.

During cholecystectomy the common duct may be injured or accidentally tied off at any level from the liver to the duodenum, or the small ductules in the gallbladder bed on the undersurface of the liver may be injured with persistent bile leakage. In addition there may be injury to the duodenum or even the head of the pancreas.

Complications

- Subhepatic Collections
  These are pools of blood, bile, or pus, under the liver and will require drainage.
- Hemorrhage
  Disturbance of the clotting mechanism causing hemorrhage during and following operation. This may occur in patients with obstructive jaundice, and is due to failure of the intestinal absorption of Vitamin K when bile is absent from the bowel. (This vitamin is required for normal blood clotting).
- Bile Peritonitis
  This may occur if bile leaks into the general abdominal cavity following surgery. Strangely, although large quantities of bile in the general cavity may produce severe surgical shock, it is not uncommon for such cases to reveal no evidence of shock or sepsis, even with five or more litres of bile in the abdomen.
- Bile Fistula
  This occurs when there is continued external drainage of bile. It may be from a bile duct, with persistent blockage by stone or stricture, or from an opening in the duodenum that was employed at surgery to obtain access the lower end of the bile duct. This opening is sutured towards the end of the operation but may reopen during the postoperative period.
- Problems with Bile Duct Drainage Tubes
  These include kinking, displacement, and retraction of the tubes, producing obstruction or leakage. The interior of the drainage tube may also become obstructed with blood clot or thick, semisolid bile. Sometimes the tube is too tightly sutured in place or is too inflexible to be remove in the usual fashion.
- *Postoperative Jaundice*
  This is a condition in which the patient's eyes and skin turn yellow due to the presence of bile pigments in the tissues. It may be due to injury of the bile duct system at operation, or retention of a stone in the bile duct following surgery. Another possibility is that of jaundice caused by *halothane*, used in general anesthesia, which may produce liver damage.
- *Postoperative Pancreatitis*
  This is an acute inflammation of the pancreas, which produces abdominal pain, fever, jaundice, and specific chemical changes in the

blood). It is caused by a blockage of the outflow of the powerful digestive juices produced by that organ, due to a stone or swelling.

OPERATIONS ON THE PANCREAS AND SPLEEN

The pancreas is a digestive organ, lying horizontally behind the stomach. It produces a highly alkaline digestive juice which is capable of digesting proteins, carbohydrates and fats. This juice is discharged into the duodenum via the pancreatic duct. The pancreas also contains clusters of *islet cells*, special cells that produce insulin (and other metabolic hormones), which controls carbohydrate metabolism and is secreted into the bloodstream.

The pancreas is divided anatomically into the "head, neck, body, and tail." The head is on the right side and the common bile duct descends through it to enter the duodenum at the same place as the pancreatic duct. The remainder of the pancreas is to the left of the head and is not involved with the bile ducts, although a stone at the lower end of the common bile duct may obstruct the pancreatic duct.

The main indications for surgery on the pancreas are cancer, *pseudocyst*, fistula, and *islet cell* tumours which cause low blood sugar. Other indications (other than trauma) are removal of all or part of the pancreas in operations that are primarily for cancer of the stomach or upper colon.

Complications

- *Pancreatic Fistula*
  This is a discharging channel between the pancreas and the skin. and can occur with any surgery of the pancreas. It is particularly troublesome because the pancreatic enzymes which are discharged onto the skin are those which produce protein digestion, thus keeping the fistula tract from healing and even causing the tract to enlarge. In persistent fistulas secondary nutritional problems may occur. Aside from operative incision of the pancreas, the commonest cause of fistula is external trauma, as in vehicular accidents. Such fistulas are especially prone to occur following biopsy of the pancreas and surgeons have therefore been increasingly reluctant to perform this

diagnostic operative procedure, especially since the microscopy results are rather unreliable. One of the problems the surgeon faces in attempting to avoid the development of pancreatic fistula is the fact that even the most careful suturing of the pancreas may produce a fistula.
- *Pancreatic Pseudocyst*
  This is a condition in which large balloon-like collections of fluid may develop in relation to this digestive organ, producing abdominal swelling and pain. It may follow any injury or inflammation of the pancreas, and may be a complication of stones in the pancreatic ducts. A common cause is the presence of alcoholic pancreatitis. Such cysts may grow to huge proportions and are best drained into the stomach or small intestine to produce a relatively harmless internal fistula.

CANCER OF THE PANCREAS

When this occurs in the head of the gland it may compress or block the common bile duct, with the production of progressive jaundice and the intolerable symptom of severe generalized itching. These problems do not occur with cancer of the remaining gland and, therefore, diagnosis is made much later.

The operation for removal of pancreatic cancer is called the
WHIPPLE PROCEDURE

This extensive and complex operation has a low cure rate and a high complication rate, but the alternative is progressive deterioration and death.
The operation consists of removal of all or part of the pancreas along with the gallbladder, the duodenum and (usually) the adjacent portion of the stomach. The common bile duct, stomach and remaining portion of the pancreas (if any) are anastomosed to the jejunum. Some type of fistula occurs in up to 20 percent of these cases.

Complications

- Hemorrhage
  This may be quite massive if major veins are torn in separating the pancreatic head from the underlying vessels. Gastrointestinal bleed-

ing may also occur postoperatively and may even require reoperation to seek and secure the bleeding vessel.
- Biliary Fistula
  This occurs uncommonly, mainly as the result of leakage at the anastomosis between the common bile duct and upper end of the small intestine.
- Gastric Fistula
  This occurs as the result of leakage at the anastomosis between the stomach and the jejunum.
- Postoperative Stricture of the Common Bile Duct
  This may occur during the postoperative period and produce a progressive jaundice which may be mistaken for recurrent or residual cancer.
- Duodenal Fistula
  This may occur with any incision of the duodenum during the course of pancreatic surgery. If the fistula persists, it leads to serious nutritional problems that compound the hazards. The management of this complication is extremely complex and presents a major challenge to the surgeon.
- General Peritonitis
  This complication only occurs as the result of inadequate drainage following pancreatic surgery. It may also occur as a result of intestinal gangrene due to impaired blood supply.
- Localized Abscesses
  These may occur under the diaphragm, under the liver, or behind the stomach (or gastric remnant). They may result from pockets of peritonitis which become shut off from the general cavity.
- *Mesenteric Thrombosis*
  Any of the major veins (and sometimes even the arteries) may clot up during or following pancreatic resection, especially the Whipple procedure. It should be remembered that the thrombosis could be the result of the malignancy rather than the operation itself. A result of such thrombosis is gangrene of the bowel, either limited or extensive.
- Liver Failure
  This may result from damage to the liver's blood supply during surgery, or from persistent obstructive jaundice (bile duct obstruction) where the possibility of pancreatic cancer is not considered until late. In the presence of alcoholic pancreatitis, there may also be an associated alcoholic cirrhosis of the liver, which will produce liver failure as a hazard of pancreatic surgery.

- Kidney Failure
  This is most likely to occur in the elderly, especially where there is a history of preexisting renal impairment. Predisposing causes include surgical shock due to the magnitude of the operation and blood loss, transfusion reaction, dehydration, postoperative sepsis, and the administration of antibiotics that are toxic to the kidneys. In cases complicated by liver failure there may be associated renal impairment as part of what has been called the *hepatorenal syndrome*.
- Gastric Ulcer (or Marginal Ulcer at the Junction with Jejunum)
  This may occur if most of the stomach is left in the Whipple procedure, and can be minimized by resecting the distal part of the stomach, or by avoiding incorrect techniques of anastomosis which divert the bile and pancreatic juice away from the gastric outlet. Such ulcers may bleed or perforate.
- Diabetes
  In addition to the digestive functions of the pancreas, with enzymes that digest fats, carbohydrates, and proteins, there is the secretion of insulin by the islet cells in the pancreas. Thus, when that organ is removed, not only is the digestion impaired but the drop in insulin production may cause the onset of diabetes. This is a far less severe type of diabetes than the type which arises spontaneously, and the danger of overtreatment with insulin administration is actually greater than that of excessive blood sugar levels.
- Long Term Nutritional Defects
  Total removal of the pancreas causes increased loss of fat in the stool, with diarrhea and protein loss. This condition is made worse when the resection includes a portion of the stomach and all of the duodenum. Even when a portion of the pancreas is left in place and implanted into the small intestine there may be stenosis of the pancreatic duct which will produce similar effects to those of total pancreatectomy.

PALLIATIVE SURGERY TO RELIEVE JAUNDICE AND SEVERE ITCHING

This is done in cases of advanced, inoperable cancer, and consists of bypassing the gallbladder or common bile duct into the jejunum. Sometimes a gastric bypass to the jejunum has to be done at the same time.

SPLENECTOMY

The spleen is a solid organ that is situated between the left side of the stomach and the left kidney. Its main function is as a part of the immune and *lymphoid* system and its structure resembles that of the lymph nodes. Besides producing specialised white blood cells, it destroys "outworn" blood *platelets*, which are an essential element in the normal clotting mechanism, as well as aging red blood cells. In addition, it breaks up the released hemoglobin. Another function is that of acting as a blood-storing organ which can empty itself into the circulation in emergency situations.

Removal of the spleen is performed for major rupture of that organ, where effective repair is impossible, and for various blood disorders that are associated with conditions that interfere with or alter the spleen's normal functions.

Complications

- Hemorrhage
  This is more likely to occur when the spleen is very large very adherent. It may also occur when the splenic vessels are very friable and do not retain their ligatures, sutures or vascular clips. Postoperative hemorrhage may be severe enough to be life-threatening.
- Pancreatic Fistula
  Because of the proximity of the pancreatic tail to the point where the blood vessels enter and leave the spleen, some degree of injury to the pancreas may occur during splenectomy, and fistula may result.
- Gastric Fistula
  This may occur due to inadvertent injury to the upper portion of the stomach or to the short vessels in that region, where the spleen is closely tied to the stomach.
- Sepsis
  Infection of the space which was occupied by the spleen may progress to the formation of a *subphrenic abscess*, a collection of pus below the diaphragm.
- Lung Complications
  These are more likely to occur in cases of splenic trauma, as in road accidents, where there may be accompanying injury to the lower left chest, with or without fractured ribs. Collapse of the lung (*atelectasis*),

usually confined to the lower lobe, may then be followed by pneumonia.
- Thrombosis
  The spleen is sometimes removed in conditions where there is an excessive destruction of blood platelets, which are essential to the normal clotting of blood. If the level of these platelets rises too high following splenectomy, the result may be a tendency towards thrombosis, particularly in the veins.
- Subsequent Infections
  Because the spleen is involved in the body's immunological system, its removal may render the patient susceptible to certain infections, of which pneumonia and meningitis are the commonest.

CHAPTER 10

Thyroid Operations and Other Types of Neck Surgery

EXCISION OF THE THYROID GLAND (*THYROIDECTOMY*)

This gland, which produces *thyroxin*, the hormone which regulates the rate of metabolism throughout the body, has two lobes, one on each side of the larynx, connected by a short *isthmus*.

The operation used to be done mostly for an excessive production of the hormone, resulting in thyroid enlargement, weight loss, bulging eyes, sweating and palpitations. This condition is called *Grave's Disease or thyrotoxicosis*. Nowadays these cases are mostly treated medically, especially with radiactive iodine, and without surgery. Most thyroid excisions today are done for lumps in the gland—which may be cancerous—and for enlargements (*goitres*) which may be generalised or lumpy, and may press on the larynx and upper trachea. Surgery of the thyroid gland involves dissection of small blood vessels and nerves which are prone to injury.

Complications

- Postoperative Bleeding
  This may produce an enlarging hematoma under the thyroid suture line and if drainage is inadequate, compression of the tracheal airway may ensue and will cause death unless promptly relieved. Sometimes the bleeding occurs at a deeper level and may be missed, but any type of respiratory difficulty should raise a suspicion of possible deep bleeding in the neck's *tissue planes* (layers).

- Air Embolism
  This complication only occurs if massive amounts of air are permitted to enter an opening in one of the major neck veins in the presence of marked negative venous pressure (acting like a vacuum) at the point of entry.
- Edema of the Larynx
  Edema is the name given to soft tissue swelling due to accumulation of fluid in the tissue spaces. This serious complication is usually amenable to treatment without *tracheostomy* (an artificial opening into the trachea and insertion of an airway tube, used to overcome laryngeal obstruction).
- Nerve Injury
  There are two nerves on each side of the thyroid gland that may be injured during the operation. Such injury may lead to anything from hoarseness to complete loss of voice. Bilateral nerve injury may cause immediate postoperative respiratory difficulty.
- *Thyroid Storm*
  In those cases where the thyroidectomy is being performed for excessive thyroid activity, this acute hyperthyroid crisis may come on during the early postoperative period. It is characterized by acute fever, rapid pulse rate, nausea, vomiting, diarrhea, and mental confusion. With the reduced number of operations for hyperthyroidism, and the correct preoperative management of these patients, the complication of thyroid storm is now less commonly seen.
- Hypothyroidism (*Myxedema*)
  This is a syndrome of reduced thyroid activity which may follow removal of a major portion of the thyroid gland. It is characterized by weight gain, dry skin and loss of hair, sluggishness, intolerance to cold, and constipation.
- Calcium Depletion
  This complication, which is known as *hypocalcemia*, is characterized by numbness and tingling, muscle cramps, and severe spasms of the hands and feet. Although this may be due to hormonal readjustments caused by removal of thyroid activity, it may be the result of damage or removal of the *parathyroids*, small glands which lie in close proximity to the thyroid, and which control calcium metabolism.
- Cosmetic Complications
  These include keloid formation in the scar, simple hypertrophy of the scar, depression of the scar with adherence to the underlying muscle, and asymmetry of the scar. In the female patient these complications can be most distressing.

- Complications of Surgery for *Substernal Goitre*
  This is a condition in which the goitre is situated behind the upper end of the breastbone, and where difficult dissection may endanger some of the adjacent major structures.
- Injury to the esophagus
- Pneumothorax
  This occurs when there is injury to the *pleura*, the membrane which lines the cavity of the chest. Any injury to the pleura allows air to enter the cavity and compress the lung in a condition known as *pneumothorax*.
- Lymph Fistula
  Another structure that may be damaged in this operation is the major duct carrying lymph to the venous outflow; this can lead to the formation of a lymph fistula.

OPERATIONS ON THE *PARATHYROID GLANDS*

These are performed for conditions in which there is excessive production of the parathyroid hormone, either due to hypertrophy or tumour of these glands. The parathyroid glands, four in number, lie behind the lobes of the thyroid gland.

Complications

- *Hypocalcemia* (Lowered Levels of Calcium in the Blood).
  This may be due to depletion of the parathyroid hormone, as well as the various small blood vessel injuries which may occur with both thyroidectomy and parathyroidectomy.

OPERATIONS FOR CANCER OF THE HEAD AND NECK

Complications

These are related to the important structures which may be damaged during complex and difficult dissections.

- Hemorrhage
  This may be profuse if there is an inadvertent tear to the main jugular vein.
- Hematoma
  In the absence of adequate drainage, the persistence of smaller degrees of bleeding may lead to the formation of hematomas in the soft tissues.
- Obstruction of Airways
  This may be due to blockage of the anesthetic tubes carrying oxygen and anesthetic gases to the lungs. It may also be due to dislodgement of the endotracheal tube or blockage with thick mucus or bloodclot. Postoperative airway obstruction may be due to swelling of the soft tissues in the mouth, throat, larynx, tissue planes of the neck, and pressure by hematoma.
- Delayed Aspiration
  This may be due to disturbance of the normal closure of the *epiglottis* (a flap below the back of the tongue) and vocal cords during swallowing.
- Air Embolism, Pneumothorax, and Lymph Fistula
  These are as described for thyroidectomy.
- Edema of the Face
  Contributing factors are the reaction to extensive facial dissections, venous obstruction, and lymphatic obstruction. It may be severe enough to cause airway obstruction.
- Increased Intracranial Pressure
  This may occur with operations that remove the main jugular vein, especially in bilateral removal of lymphnodes of the neck for cancer.
- Infection
  This can be combatted with correct drainage and antibiotics, but it should be remembered that fever of noninfective origin may result from extensive dissections in this region. If sepsis extends downwards into the chest it may set up a dangerous complication known as *mediastinitis*, in which the infection involves the soft tissues around the heart and great vessels.
- Nerve Complications
  There are many sensory nerves in this region which may be damaged during this type of surgery, resulting in temporary or permanent sensory disturbance. There are also motor nerves which may be damaged, especially the nerve to the shoulder elevators in radical removal

of lymph nodes for cancer. More importantly the facial nerve may be damaged during removal of the parotid salivary gland (the "mumps gland") for tumour. This will result in permanent facial paralysis, whereas temporary paralysis may result from temporary pressure or traction on the nerve during dissection.

- Death of the Skin Flaps

    This occurs with large flaps that are poorly supplied with blood vessels and is more likely to occur where infection, hematoma, or malnutrition are present. These skin flaps are fashioned by the surgeon and separated from the underlying structures in order to obtain wide exposure of the operative field and to obtain coverage of open areas at the end of the operation.

- Postoperative Malnutrition

    This may result from difficulties in eating and drinking which follow some of these operative procedures.

CHAPTER 11

Operations on the Heart and Lungs

SURGERY OF THE HEART

Most heart operations today are for blockage of the coronary arteries and for the replacement of defective heart valves with artificial valves.

In order to enable the surgeon to perform open heart surgery it is necessary to bypass the circulating blood away from the heart and lungs by means of a special pump and oxygen-provider, namely a heart-lung bypass.

Temporary Heart-Lung Bypass

A procedure known as the *cardiopulmonary bypass* provides a maintained blood circulation which excludes the heart's cavities and is carried on outside the body, *extracorporeal perfusion*. This is done by a series of tubes and a special device known as a **pump oxygenator** which keeps the blood circulating and oxygenates it without the blood traversing the lungs. It is a highly complex procedure, with the possibility of technical surgical mishaps and disturbances of blood chemistry as well as the causing of organic disorders.

Complications

- Injuries to Major Vessels. These may occur during insertion of the tubes, known as *cannulas*, and must be carefully guarded against.
- Oxygen Deficiency
  This may result from underperfusion or overdilution of the blood with other fluids.
- Flow Obstructions
  These may occur due to kinking of the cannulas or conduction tubes,

even by a member of the surgical team inadvertently standing on one of the tubes.
- Kidney Malfunction
  This may be due to underperfusion.
- Red Blood Cell Destruction
  This condition, known as *hemolysis*, is caused by abnormal flow patterns in the circulating blood as it passes through the various chambers or from transfusion reaction and will contribute to renal failure.
- Other complications, such as acidification of the blood and specific electrolyte disturbances, microemboli, and air embolism, are largely preventable by skilful management.

GENERAL Complications OF CARDIAC SURGERY

- Hemorrhage
  This may be due to damage to the heart or major vessels, to imperfect suture lines, or to clotting deficiencies. It may result in death during surgery or postoperatively.
- Heart Block
  This may occur as the result of sutures that inadvertently include portions of the electrical conduction systems that regulate the heart rhythm. It is most likely to occur during the insertion of artificial heart valves.
- *Peripheral Embolism*
  This is a condition where clots in the heart or arteries are circulated away from the heart and lungs towards the brain, the limbs or various organs in the body. It may occur in situations where arterial plaques (see Chapter 16) are dislodged, especially from diseased heart valves. It may also originate from clots in the proximal chamber on the right side of the heart (*atrial thrombi*).
- *Air Embolism*
  This is most likely to occur in those operations involving entry into the heart chambers, and may impair cardiac filling and emptying or produce strokes by entry into the brain circulation by way of the carotid arteries.
- Respiratory Complications
  These are the same as may occur with most chest surgery but are more likely to occur in those patients whose heart condition has already produced some degree of respiratory insufficiency.
- Infection
  This may produce a mediastinitis or even a bone infection of the

sternum. Infection may also reach the chest cavity on either side and produce an *empyema* (see P.104). A particular hazard is the involvement of a valve replacement in an infective process (because it is almost impossible to clear up sepsis in artificial implants that remain in the body).

Complications of coronary bypass operations

- Problems with the Vein Graft
  This graft is taken from the thigh and inserted between the aorta and the coronary artery beyond the blockage. It may be too long and become kinked; it may be too short and place tension on the suture line. It may become obstructed through kinking or twisting, or through being incorrectly inserted with the valves pointing the wrong way. It may also bleed through tiny side branch stumps, or minute tears.
- Problems with the Aorta
  These are due to calcification or excessive friability of this major vessel at the level of its arch (the first portion) and may cause either leakage at the suture line, compression of the anastomosis, or embolism.
- *Myocardial Infarction*
  This term means that the blood supply to part of the heart muscle is cut off, causing that muscle to lose its function, with possible fatal results. It may occur either during or following cardiac surgery.
- Postoperative *Arrhythmia* (Irregular Heartbeat)
  This is most commonly of the atrial type—affecting the upper chambers of the heart—and is amenable to medication. Rarely, electroconversion of arrhythmia is required (by applying electric shocks to the heart through the chest wall).
- Pulmonary Embolism
  Fortunately this is now a rare complication. It may occur if the patient has had a cardiac catheter inserted and then remains in bed waiting for coronary bypass.
- Neurological Complications
  These are commonest in patients with a history of stroke and those with evidence of carotid artery disease. Severe stroke or death may occur as a result of cerebral embolism.
  Aside from the brain, other neurological complications may occur. These include injury to the nerve to the diaphragm, the nerve to the larynx (on the left side), and even the nerve trunks in the axilla.

68   *Informed Consent to Surgery*

- Disease of the Vein Graft
  After the first few successful years following coronary bypass the vein graft may develop the same changes of hardening of the arteries, arteriosclerosis, as those present in the coronary and arteries.

SURGERY OF THE LUNGS

The main operation performed on the lung is done mostly for certain types of cancer; it may be partial or total lung removal and is called *pulmonary resection*. Complications may occur during surgery, such as injury to blood vessels or to the esophagus, and difficulties with closure of the bronchial stump. There may also be difficulty in expanding the remaining portion of the lung after partial resection, due to blood or thick mucus in the air channels, or an incorrectly positioned endotracheal tube. The modern tendency is towards fewer total pulmonary resections in favour of lesser, lobar, segmental, or wedge resections.

Complications

- Bleeding from the Chest Wall
  This comes mainly from separated adhesions and generally does not require reoperation, unless it persists when the clotting mechanism is functioning normally. The amount of bleeding is easily monitored because of the drainage tubes that are routinely inserted in the chest cavity at the end of partial resections. In total resections, drainage tubes are not used in the chest cavity, and excessive amounts of fluid or air are removed by needle aspiration. This is done in order to keep the mediastinum from shifting towards the opposite side (because of the difference in the air pressure in the two chest cavities).
- Hemorrhage from the Major Blood Vessels
  This is probably due to ligatures slipping off the main pulmonary vessels or their branches. Reexploration is urgent and mandatory.
- Lung Collapse
  This complication (*atelectasis*) is generally due to collection of mucous secretions in the bronchial tree, and is usually partial rather than complete.
- Air Leaks
  These are easily diagnosed by the appearance of copious air bubbles

in the drainage bottles following surgery and may represent a raw area on the surface of the remaining lung, or a bronchial leak if persistent and associated with major lung collapse. If the air escapes into the soft tissues, the condition of *subcutaneous or mediastinal emphysema* may result. This syndrome is characterized by swelling of the face, neck, and upper torso, with a crackling sensation on pressing the skin. X-rays will reveal air in the subcutaneous areas and mediastinum.

- Cardiac Distortion

  Displacement or torsion of the heart may occur with complete removal of the lung, in those cases where it becomes necessary to open the envelope that surrounds the heart, (called the *pericardium*). It may cause shock and even cardiac arrest shortly after surgery.

- Gangrene of the Lung

  This may occur if one of the remaining lobes of the lung becomes twisted and shuts off its own blood supply. It is most likely to affect the right middle lobe following resection of the upper lobe.

- Bronchial Leakage

  Major air leakage after the first ten postoperative days is highly suggestive of a *bronchopleural fistula*, an open passage between the bronchial stump and the chest cavity.

- Esophagopleural Fistula

  Pulmonary resections are usually accompanied by lymph node removal in the region of the large bloodvessels between the lungs. When this is done on the right side there is danger of injury to the blood supply of the esophagus, followed by the formation of fistula between the gullet and the chest cavity.

- Nerve Injury

  On the left side, the nerve to the larynx may be injured, causing persistent hoarseness.

- Infection

  Empyema is the name given to a collection of pus in the chest cavity (pleural space). It may occur after any type of lung resection where there is a persistent space between the residual lung and the chest wall, or no lung on that side (total resection), and retained blood or fluid secretions become infected. Fever may be the only clinical sign. Wound infection should be diagnosed early and treated vigorously because of the danger of empyema. (Empyema may also occur with any surgery of the chest).

CHAPTER 12

Operations on the Arterial System

Preamble

Arteriosclerosis or *Atherosclerosis* are the two medical names for so-called "hardening of the arteries." The abreviation *ASD* will be used in subsequent reference to this condition (the D is for disease).

ASD is a degenerative process in which deposits of cholesterol and related fatty substances are formed on the interior of arteries. They may cause thrombosis in the artery, blockage of the artery, either partial or complete, and weakening of the arterial wall, with possible development of aneurysm. The soft, mushy material of ASD deposits or plaques may become calcified, and produce the so-called "eggshell" artery, which is difficult to incise or suture during vascular surgery.

SURGERY OF THE ABDOMINAL AORTA

The abdominal aorta is the continuation of the thoracic aorta and extends from the diaphragm to the top of the pelvis where it branches into two common iliac arteries.

There are two main situations for which aortic surgery is indicated. One is *aortic occlusion and the other is aortic aneurysm.*

Aortic Occlusion

This is due in most instances to the progressive deposition of plaques (due to ASD), with or without calcification, causing narrowing and then obstruction of the channel.

The usual operation for this condition is a bypass graft, usually of dacron fabric tubing. This is inserted into the aorta below the vessels to the kidneys and into the common iliac arteries below, or into the main arteries below the groin, known as the *common femoral arteries*. Another type of surgery which is sometimes done for this condition, particularly in the terminal aorta and iliac arteries, is *endarterectomy*. This consists of opening up the arterial channel, dissecting off the plaque material from the interior, cleaning it out and then suturing up the incision in the artery.

Abdominal Aortic Aneurysm
In this condition, ASD of the aorta below the diaphragm causes a weakening of the arterial wall and a balloon-like dilatation of the vessel (*aneurysm*), with increasing danger of rupture.

The operation consists of opening the ballooned segment between special noncrushing clamps. The large indwelling clot is removed and a graft of knitted (sometimes woven) dacron is sutured to the cut end of the aorta above and to the bifurcation below (sometimes to the common iliacs or the common femoral arteries below the groin).

Complications of aortic surgery

- Injury to the major veins
  These are adjacent to and may be adherent to the abdominal aorta and its bifurcation. Such injuries during surgery may cause serious or catastrophic hemorrhage.
- Injury to the *Ureters*
  These are the tubes leading from the kidneys to the urinary bladder. They may be injured due to adherence of the ureter to the wall of an aortic aneurysm, or during dissection in the region of the iliac vessels, and may cause leakage of urine into the abdominal cavity, to eventual loss of the kidney, or infection of the graft.
- Blood Clotting Below the Aortic Clamp
  This must be guarded against in all arterial surgery and may, if uncorrected, lead to blockage of the graft with unsatisfactory flow or the possibility of producing embolism.
- Serious Leakage at the Suture Lines
  This may require additional sutures but often reponds to gentle pressure over a dry pack.

- Kinking of the Graft
  This may occur if the graft is too long, producing turbulent or obstructed flow.
- Embolism
  This may be due to the flushing of ASD deposits into the distal arteries.
- Obstruction at the Lower Anastomosis
  This may occur due to ASD of the artery to which the graft has been joined.
- *Dissection* of the Arterial Wall
  This term refers to fragmentation of the interior of the distal vessel, which causes separation of the artery's layers.
- Damage to the Blood Supply of the Spinal Cord
  This complication causes paralysis of the lower limbs. It is more common with aneurysms involving the upper levels of the aorta.
- Damage to the Blood Supply of the Left Colon
  This may occur during the initial surgical dissection on the left side of the aorta.
- Injury to the Duodenum
  This may occur during the dissection around the upper end of the abdominal aorta or when suturing the covering peritoneal membrane over the upper anastomosis.
- Postoperative Abdominal Distension
  This may produce respiratory difficulties and wound disruption. Insertion of a nasogastric tube in such cases is preferable to tube gastrostomy in order to avoid the hazard of graft infection.
- Graft Infection
  This is a very serious complication and means that the graft will have to be removed and a secondary bypass performed.

FEMOROPOPLITEAL BYPASS

This operation involves the insertion of a graft between the common femoral artery above and the *popliteal* artery below the knee. The graft that is usually employed is a segment of superficial vein in the thigh, known as the *long saphenous vein*, or a thin, pliable material known as *goretex*.

Complications

- Stenosis at Either of the Anastomoses
  Narrowing may occur where the graft joins the artery
- Twisting of the Graft
  This must be guarded against during surgery.
- Persistent Bleeding
  This may occur from one or more holes in the vein graft or the stumps of small branches.
- Postoperative Thrombosis of the Graft
- Postoperative Embolism
  Small clots from the operative area may shift downwards and obstruct a lower artery.
- Graft infection
  As pointed out previously, infection in artificial implant material is very hard to clear up and the graft has to be removed in such cases.
- False Aneurysm
  A late ballooning at the site of an anastomosis may occur due to weakening of the artery where it is sutured.

CAROTID ENDARTERECTOMY

The *common carotid* artery is the major artery in the neck that supplies the brain and face and various important structures in the head and neck. At the level of the angle of the lower jaw, it divides into the internal and external branches, with the internal division proceeding up into the skull to supply the brain.

ASD plaques in the internal carotid artery may produce increasing stenosis of the vessel or emboli to the brain from an ulcerating plaque, with the production of transient strokes.

Carotid endarterectomy is an operation to remove the plaque and leave a smooth-walled interior of the artery.

Complications

- Failure to Maintain the Patient's Blood Pressure during the operation—resulting in stroke.
- Nerve Injury
  Damage to the nerve that supplies the muscles of the tongue, causing

paralysis of the tongue, is usually temporary.
- Embolism to the Brain
  This may be produced by failure to prevent upward flow of plaque fragments during operative dissection or by the insertion of a temporary shunt. It may also occur if the open vessel is inadequately flushed clean prior to suture.
- Persistent Bleeding at the Suture Line
  This may be due to inadequate reversal of anticoagulant. The patient is given an intravenous dose of an anticlotting agent before applying the arterial clamps. At the end of the procedure an intravenous injection of reversing agent is given to restore normal clotting.
- Hematoma Formation
  This is usually caused by inadequate suction-drainage of the wound.
- Early Postoperative Hypertension
  This may be quite severe in the recovery room and should be carefully controlled by judicious use of intravenous antihypertensive agents. Otherwise renewed bleeding may occur, with an enlarging hematoma or increased blood drainage.

CHAPTER 13

Other Operations for Blood Vessel Disorders

SURGERY FOR THE *THORACIC OUTLET SYNDROME*

This is a set of symptoms and signs due to narrowing of the space between the collar bone and the uppermost ribs. There may be significant compression of the nerve trunks, the arteries, or the veins which pass through this space, on their way from the lower neck to the axilla and then to the upper limb.

The operation, which is done when other methods of management (such as physiotherapy and weight-loss) fail, consists of removing the first rib and sometimes an extra rib in the lower neck, in order to relieve the pressure in the closed space. It is usually performed through the axilla.

Complications

- Hemorrhage
  This may be due to damage of the vessels during the dissection, during division of the rib with bone-cutters, or to bone *spicules* (little spikes) on the ends of the severed bone, if these are not carefully smoothed.
- Nerve Damage
  This may occur in the same way as vascular injury, or it may be due to overstretching of the nerve trunks when the surgeon's assistant forcibly elevates the arm to facilitate the surgical access to the axillary depths.

- *Pneumothorax*
  Air enters the chest cavity if the pleura over the apex of the lung is entered during surgery. Lung collapse may follow.
- Wound Infection
  In obese patients, those with excessive sweating, and those with recurrent axillary infections, there will be a higher incidence of this complication unless preventive measures are employed.

THE OPERATION OF *SYMPATHECTOMY*

This is the name given to a surgical procedure involving the removal of certain portions of the nervous system, called the *sympathetic nervous system*, that control nonvoluntary functions.

These include such functions as the muscular activity controlling the pupil of the eye, the bronchial tree, the digestive tract, and the urinary tract, as well as the secretions of glandular tissue, and the activity of the heart and blood vessels.

The leading indications for such operations are conditions of excessive arterial spasm causing serious impairment of the blood flow. There are two main diseases in this category.

The first of these is *Raynaud's disease*, a condition which is commonest in young women. It affects the digits, usually in the hands, and the symptoms of pain and colour changes may be brought on by exposure to cold or emotional upset. There is no associated disease of the vessel wall and no involvement of the larger limb arteries. It may progress to ulceration and gangrene of the digits. The condition may affect non-smokers.

The second of these disorders is *Buerger's disease*, commonest in relatively young men. It, too, affects the digits and may produce similar symptoms, but it is always associated with addiction to cigarettes. It is often preceded by and associated with phlebitis in the limb, and leads to a process of gangrene which may extend up the limb. The vascular walls reveal an inflammation and thickening that is quite different from *ASD*.

DORSAL (THORACIC) SYMPATHECTOMY

This is done for severe *vasospastic* disease (spasm of the vessels, mainly the small arteries) of the upper limb that does not respond to nonoperative methods.

Complications

- Pneumothorax
  Air in the chest cavity may occur accidentally even if the surgical approach is outside the pleural lining of the chest. It is more likely to occur as the result of an intrapleural approach to the upper dorsal sympathetic chain, through the chest wall.
- Damage to the Axillary Nerves and Vessels
  This is most likely to occur with a surgical approach through the axilla, but can usually be avoided with appropriate care.
- *Horner's Syndrome*
  This is due to removal of too much sympathetic nerve chain at the upper end of the dorsal sympathectomy. It is characterized by constriction of the pupil, drooping of the upper eyelid, recession of the eye (which looks smaller), and dryness of the face on the side of the operation.

LUMBAR SYMPATHECTOMY

This is done for severe vasospastic conditions of the lower limbs which do not respond to nonoperative methods such as medication, avoidance of cigarettes and protection from exposure to cold.

Complications

- Hemorrhage
  This may occur during surgery, due to tearing of the veins that cross the sympathetic chain.
- Excessive Dryness and Cracking of the Skin
  This is due to removal of the sympathetic nerves that are responsible for causing increased sweating.
- *Neuralgia*
  This painful condition may be quite persistent following this operation and may represent minor injury to some of the neighbouring nerves. It is usually self-limiting.

- Impotence in the Male
  This may occur if removal of the upper end of the sympathetic chain is carried too high. It is due to interference with the nerve control of penile erection. This may be permanent.
- Abdominal Distension
  This is due to paralytic ileus and should not occur with careful dissection alongside the vertebrae and outside the abdominal cavity.

OPERATIONS FOR VENOUS INCOMPETENCE

This is a condition of failure of the valves in the veins to counteract the effects of gravity. The commonest visible evidence of this condition is the appearance of varicose veins in the lower limbs. These can be very large, tortuous, and disfiguring, can be prone to attacks of phlebitis, and may be complicated by incompetence of the deep veins. Severe cases can progress to chronic ulceration of the leg. Normally this venous competence is maintained by a system of valves in the veins, and by the pumping action of the calf muscles.

Mild cases do not require surgery and may be treated by suitable elastic support, avoidance of prolonged standing, and by injection techniques.

Injection treatment of varicose veins was in great vogue half a century ago but was abandoned for several good reasons. Leakage of the sclerosant solution into the deep veins destroyed the deep valvular mechanism, and leakage into the skin produced ugly discolouration or ulceration. Even with successful techniques the improvement was often short-lived, the recurrences more severe than the original condition, and the subsequent corrective surgery rendered more difficult. Despite the recent surge in the popularity of "new" injection techniques, there are still many surgeons who get the best results with surgery.

VEIN STRIPPING

This operation consists of dividing the main superficial vein of the lower limb at the level of the groin and removing that vein down to the lower ankle. It is done by means of a special stripping instrument that is passed down the vein. Sometimes the superficial vein on the back of the lower leg requires stripping, and sometimes major branch channels require division or excision. Fortunately, when this is done, the normal veins with intact valves take over the function of removed veins.

Complications

- Bleeding and Hematoma Formation
  This should be prevented by suitable elastic bandaging of the leg from toes to upper thigh, and elevation of the leg when the patient is in bed.
- Postoperative Thrombosis
  This is prevented by early mobilization of the patient. Walking is encouraged; sitting is discouraged, although it may be permitted for short periods as long as the leg is kept straight or supported on a second chair.
- Swelling of the Foot
  This is prevented by correct bandaging and rebandaging as necessary, with inclusion of the entire foot. Elastic bandaging should always be done from the toes upwards.
- Nerve Injury
  Numbness around the ankle is quite common and is due to injury to nerve fibres when the vein is stripped through the lower incision. The numbness usually clears up during the first year following surgery.
- Groin Infection
  This can be avoided by proper removal of hair from the groin area and thorough cleansing prior to surgery. After surgery, the groin incision should remain uncovered, washed three times daily with a mild antiseptic, and carefully dried. Sutures should be removed as early as possible and replaced by skin-tapes.
- Scars
  These should be minimal with correct placement of incisions.
- Residual or Recurrent Varicosities
  This is the ideal indication for injection therapy, as there is minimal danger of deep vein involvement.

THE LINTON-COCKETT PROCEDURE

This operation was devised separately by Dr. R.R.Linton in the U.S.A. and Mr. F.B. Cockett in Britain, for dealing with severe deep venous incompetence. This condition produces swelling of the leg, leathery induration of the skin, often with constriction above the ankle, dark discolouration of the skin, and progressive nonhealing ulceration.

The operation consists of a full-length incision of back of the leg from knee to ankle, incision of the fibrous envelope containing the calf muscles, and division of the several incompetent communicating veins between the superficial and deep veins.

Complications

- Hematoma
  This is prevented by correct elastic bandaging.
- Thrombosis
  This is prevented by early mobilization, although walking is avoided and foot-ankle exercises substituted instead. When the patient is lying in bed the leg should be kept at high elevation.
- Pulmonary Embolism
  If there is the slightest hint of such a condition, then intravenous anticlotting agents should be immediately commenced and the patient kept in bed.
- Necrosis of the Wound Margins
  This is more likely to occur with deep, wide, or continuous skin sutures.

Since the operation of vein stripping and related surgery for venous incompetence have received rather adverse (and unfair) criticism in recent years, the simple measures needed to avoid complications have been described in some detail.

CHAPTER 14

Urological Operations

NEPHRECTOMY

Removal of the kidney is usually performed for cancer, where the procedure is more radical, including the surrounding tissues and lymph nodes as well as the ureter. It is also performed for such destructive infections as those associated with some cases of advanced kidney stones, and tuberculosis of the kidney.

Complications

- Hemorrhage
  This is most likely to occur if the tumour has reached the renal vein, and where an attempt is made to divide this vein as close as possible to the main venous trunk (the *inferior vena cava*). A tear of the venous wall in this region may lead to catastrophic loss of blood.
- Tumour Embolism
  This may be caused by tumour material in the vein becoming dislodged by operative manipulation during nephrectomy.
- *Arteriovenous Fistula*
  This abnormal communication between artery and vein may follow mass tying, rather than individual tying, of the renal vessels in difficult kidney dissections.
- Pneumothorax
  When the kidney is very large and it is necessary to remove one or two ribs for sufficient access, the lower pleural cavity may inadvertently be entered.

- Peritonitis
  On the right side, the colon may be adherent to the kidney, especially with tuberculosis, and this may lead to accidental injury to the bowel with infection of the abdominal cavity. Alternatively, a fecal fistula may develop outside the peritoneal cavity.
- Late Postoperative Hernia
  Wound disruption of the operative incision is a less common cause than injury to nerves that supply the abdominal muscles.
- Wound Infection
  This is likely to occur with nephrectomy for an infected kidney, with inadequate drainage, and with inadequate antibiotic control.
- Kidney Failure
  Failure to check for an adequately functioning kidney on the opposite side. This complication is fatal, and inexcusible.
- Hypertension of Renal Origin
  Certain types of high blood pressure are due to an impaired arterial circulation to the kidney. If the kidney structure and function are hopelessly destroyed, the diseased organ should be removed. If there is a proven stenosis of the renal artery, then either bypass or endarterectomy may be required in appropriate cases. Complications are those of other vascular procedures as previously described.

KIDNEY TRANSPLANTATION

This is the most successful form of organ transplantion to date and owes much to the development of tissue matching techniques and to the chemical agents which suppress the natural immunity reactions.

Complications

- Immediate or Delayed Rejection
  This occurs when the immune system of the patient (the transplant recipient) attacks the tissues of the implanted kidney.
- Urinary Fistula
  This is more likely to occur when there is an anastomosis between the donor ureter and the lower end of the patient's ureter, rather than with the bladder. When it occurs it is in the early postoperative period.
- Stricture of the Lower End of the Donor Ureter
  This may occur when the donor ureter is implanted into the patient's

urinary bladder, the preferred procedure. When it occurs it is in the late postoperative period.
- Thrombosis of the Donor Vessels
  Thrombosis is more likely in the vein, but the artery may also be involved.
- Leakage at the Vascular Anastomosis
  This is usually the result of infection and may prove to be catastrophic.
- Kinking of the Anastomosed Vessels
  This and other problems with the vascular anastomosis may cause destruction of the donor kidney.
- Infection and Failure of Wound Healing
  These are more likely to occur because of the special immunosuppressive drugs (chemicals that suppress the natural immune response). These are used to safeguard the renal transplant but cancel the beneficial effects of immunity.
- Systemic Effects of the Immunosuppressive Drugs
  These include diminished resistance to infection with viruses, bacteria and fungi, as well as to the onset of malignancies.

PROSTATECTOMY

(Resection of the Prostate Gland). The commonest condition for which this operation is performed is that known as *benign prostatic hypertrophy*. This is a nonmalignant enlargement of the prostate gland, which eventually produces urinary obstruction.

OPEN SUPRAPUBIC PROSTATECTOMY

This is the oldest type of surgery for this condition and in experienced hands is a perfectly safe procedure for very large prostates. An incision is made in the central lower abdomen and the urinary bladder is opened. The hypertrophied lobe of the prostate gland is shelled out, bleeding points are ablated, usually by diathermy, and the bladder closed, with an indwelling special balloon catheter that fills the prostatic bed.

Complications

- Delayed Hemorrhage
  This usually occurs after the first week, and may produce clots in the bladder that require evacuation.
- Postoperative Incontinence of Urine
  This is nearly always temporary.

PERINEAL PROSTATECTOMY

This is done from below, with the dissection carried up between the rectum and the urethra. It works very well with certain types of prostatic enlargement.

Complications

- These are the same as above but with a lower incidence.

RETROPUBIC PROSTATECTOMY

In this procedure, also known as the Millin operation, an incision is made just above the pubis and dissection is carried out from the outside of the lower bladder. It is an improvement on the open suprapubic method.

Complications

- These are the same as above but with a lower incidence.

TRANSURETHRAL PROSTATECTOMY

Also known as a TUR, it is done without operative incision, by passing a special viewing instrument, a *resectoscope*, into the bladder. The hypertrophied prostatic lobe is resected in small strips with an electrically heated wire loop until a smooth cavity is left. Bleeding is minimized by the use of electro-cauterization. This is the commonest form of prostatectomy performed today and is best for the smaller adenomas and the fibrous prostate.

Complications

- These are the exception rather than the rule, but when they occur they are similar to the ones described for the other prostatectomies. Impotence does not occur as a result of these operations, but retrograde ejaculation of semen into the bladder is inevitable.

RADICAL PROSTATECTOMY FOR CANCER

This is a much more extensive procedure than the other types of prostatectomy and includes the seminal vesicles and the external capsule which surrounds the prostate gland. It is reserved for localized cancer before invasion of the capsule.

Complications

- Severe Hemorrhage
  This comes from the pelvic veins.
- Postoperative Urinary Fistula
  This comes from the severed prostatic portion of the urethra.
- Infection
  When this occurs it is quite severe and requires strenuous antibiotic therapy.
- Permanent Impotence
  This is an inevitable consequence of radical prostatectomy for cancer.

TOTAL CYSTECTOMY

This is a complete removal of the urinary bladder and is done for invasive cancer of the urinary bladder. There are two main types of bladder malignancies. The commoner type consists of one or more small raspberry-like growths on the interior surface; these are usually dealt with by the resectoscope. The other is the invasive type and may require total cystectomy. Prior to this procedure, it is necessary to divert the urinary flow.
(See Urinary Diversion below).

Complications

- Injury to the Pelvic Blood Vessels
- Injury to the Rectum
  This may occur if this structure is adherent to the back of the bladder.

URINARY DIVERSION

CUTANEOUS URETEROSTOMY

In this operation the ureter is brought out to the skin and drains into a bag-device. It is a temporary measure and is rarely used.

URETEROSIGMOIDOSTOMY

In this operation, also known as the "Coffey Procedure", the ureters are implanted into the sigmoid colon and the urine is evacuated periodically via the rectum. No bag or other device is worn.

Complications

- Disturbance of the Fluid-Electrolyte Balance
  This is the commonest complication, and is due to partial absorption of the urine through the bowel wall.
- Infection of the Urine
  This may require appropriate antibiotic therapy.
- Rectal Incontinence of Urine
  This occurs rarely and is due to loss of anal tone.

URETEROILEOSTOMY

This is the operation of choice, and involves the isolation of a segment of small intestine with its blood supply, called an *ileal loop*. The ureters are implanted into this ileal loop, one end of which is closed and the other brought up to the skin as an ileostomy. Drainage is into a special bag-device worn by the patient.

Complications

- These include stricture of the *ostomy opening, also known as the stoma*, and infection, which is uncommon. These second and third methods of urinary diversion carry separate risks of problems with the ureteric anastomosis. They are technical and can be largely avoided by meticulous operative technique.

SURGERY FOR *HYDROCELE OF THE TESTICLE*

This is a condition in which fluid collects progressively in the sac located inside the scrotum and which surrounds the testicle. The swelling may reach the size of a grapefruit or more before the patient seeks attention. The definitive cure of this condition is by appropriate surgery, either removal of the redundant sac-membrane or suturing the sac inside out. In the very young, and especially in infancy, this condition often communicates with a hernial sac which must be dissected up to its origin and removed.

Complications

- Scrotal Hematoma
  This is the main complication and can be prevented by accurate attention to bleeding points during surgery, and correct insertion of a drain at the close of the procedure.

SURGERY FOR UNDESCENDED TESTICLE

This condition is associated with a higher incidence of testicular cancer in later life if it remains uncorrected. It should be dealt with by corrective surgery at the earliest possible age after the patient's fourth birthday. It is usually associated with a congenital hernia.

Complications

- Excessive Traction on the *Spermatic Cord*
  This is the main complication. This excessive traction interferes with the blood supply to the testicle and causes it to atrophy. If it is impossible to bring down the testicle into the scrotum, even with two stage surgery, then the testicle should be removed. In the adult, a high lying testicle is extremely prone to injury during contact sports and sexual intercourse.

CHAPTER 15

Specific Operations on Women

SURGERY FOR BREAST CANCER

There is a good deal of confusion among surgeons as to what is the best treatment of breast cancer in women and, therefore, even greater confusion among patients with this condition. As in so many fields of surgery, what was regarded as correct in past years is regarded as wrong today, and what was regarded as wrong half a century ago—namely "Lumpectomy" or partial breast removal—is now in vogue. Nevertheless, with most experienced surgeons today, the standard operation for cancer of the breast without major spread to the lymph nodes is an operation known as "Modified Radical Mastectomy." This operation is performed where the cancer is small and mobile and there is no ulceration of the overlying skin, where preliminary biopsy confirms the presence of malignancy and investigation reveals no evidence of *metastatic* spread. This is the so-called curable stage and has the best long-term outlook. Some of the biopsy specimen is also submitted for special hormonal studies.

LUMPECTOMY

This consists of removal of the cancerous lump and what is judged to be a safe margin of normal surrounding tissue. An alternative is a partial breast removal or "quadrant resection."

Complications

- Leaving malignant tissue behind which may lead to more extensive cancer and possible spread to other areas.
- Deformity of the Breast
  If the lumpectomy is large and the breast is relatively small there will be a marked residual hollow in the breast.

MODIFIED RADICAL MASTECTOMY

This operation consists of removal of the entire breast with overlying skin and surrounding soft tissues, but without removal of the underlying muscles. In addition, the lymph nodes are removed from the axilla in order to establish the degree of malignant lymph node involvement. This helps to "stage" the cancer for correct management. This management may include radiation therapy, chemotherapy, and hormonal therapy.

Complications

- Bleeding
  Major bleeding should be controlled during surgery but oozing under the skin flaps may continue postoperatively and produce a subcutaneous hematoma on the chest wall or in the axilla. This can be avoided by adequate suction drainage.
- Seroma
  Collection of serum under the skin flaps or in the axilla. This is far commoner than hematoma and similarly avoidable.
- Breakdown of Skin Margins
  This may be caused by the flaps being too thin or by being sutured under excessive tension. This complication is worse if hematoma or seroma are also present.
- Narrowing of the Axillary Vein
  This is due to venous branches being clipped or ligated too close to the major vein in the axilla, producing a local narrowing that may cause swelling of the arm.
- Shoulder Stiffness
  This should be temporary and can be prevented by appropriate physiotherapy commencing immediately after recovery from the anesthetic.

90 *Informed Consent to Surgery*

- Scar Contracture
  This is most likely to occur if the incision is carried up into the axilla.
- Swelling of the Arm
  This is mainly due to lymphatic obstruction. It should not occur with well-performed surgery but is seen more more commonly after radiation therapy.
- Cosmetic Defect
  The absence of the breast can be very well concealed by the excellent artificial breasts available today, which are worn inside the bras. Surgical reconstruction of the breast with an artificial, implanted breast, is also available if the patient so desires. Correct placement of the mastectomy scar well below the collar bone makes it possible for the patient to wear a strapless evening gown or a swim suit with nobody the wiser.
- Effects of Associated Treatment
  (If significant axillary lymph node cancer is found, then the toxic and biological ill-effects of chemotherapy or radiation must be added to those of surgery).

CLASSICAL RADICAL MASTECTOMY

This operation has been largely replaced by the modified form. It includes the removal of the pectoral muscles behind the breast, and is usually reserved for those cases where the cancer is located deeply and is in contact with the underlying muscle.

Complications

- Nerve Injuries
  These may involve the nerve to the deep chest muscle which keeps the shoulder blade against the ribs when the arm pushes forwards against resistance. The nerve to the back muscle which is used in the downward push of the arm against resistance, may also be damaged.
- Hematoma and Seroma, Breakdown of Wound Margins, Shoulder Stiffness, Scar Contractures, and Axillary Vein Narrowing. These are more common than with the modified procedure.
- Cosmetic Defect
  In particular there is a noticeable hollow below the outer end of the collar bone. Reconstruction and implantation of an artificial breast are more difficult and less satisfactory.

- Swelling of the Arm
  This is mainly due to lymphatic obstruction. Although it is more probable with radiation therapy, it is commoner with the classical radical mastectomy than with the modified procedure.

HYSTERECTOMY

Total abdominal hysterectomy is the standard type of removal of the uterus. It is performed much less frequently in recent years, and for a stringent set of clinical and pathological indications, especially cancer of the uterine lining. Simultaneous removal of the tubes and ovaries should not be done simply because the patient is over the age of forty, but for disease that involves these structures, and for all cases of uterine cancer.

Complications

- Hemorrhage
  This may be due at operation to arterial or venous bleeding and is more troublesome when the uterus is very large or very adherent to adjacent tissues or when the pelvis is unduly small and deep. Post-operatively it may occur due to slipping of a suture or vascular clip.
- Injury to the Ureter
  In difficult hysterectomies the ureter may be inadvertently cut or sutured. If recognized, it can be repaired at once.
- Injury to the Bladder
  This may occur if the bladder is inadvertently opened during the operative entry to the lower abdomen, or during separation from the uterine body or cervix, or from the upper vagina. The important thing is to recognize and repair the injury without undue delay.
- Intestinal Injury
  This may occur during operative entry into the lower abdomen when the intestine is adherent to the abdominal wall, or even to the skin if there is an operative scar in that region. It may also occur when the bowel is adherent to the uterus or pelvic floor. Failure to visualize and repair such injury will result in peritonitis.
- Internal Fistula
  This is more likely to occur when this operation, (but more especially a radical operation), is performed for cancer. Such a fistula may be between small intestine and vagina, rectum and vagina, or small intestine and skin.

- Urinary Infection
  This may occur in the absence of injury or fistula and is one of the hazards of prolonged catheter drainage.
- *Retroperitoneal Infection*
  This may occur in the back of the pelvis, behind the peritoneal layer and therefore ouside the abdominal cavity. It may begin in a retroperitoneal hematoma and progress to an abscess.
- Painful or Difficult Intercourse
  This may be due to shortening or narrowing of the vagina and lack of vaginal moisture, but is often due to psychological inhibition.

CHAPTER 16

Two Other Common Operations

Orthopedic operations and neurosurgery are outside the scope of this book but, because of their frequency, total hip joint replacement and surgery for displaced intervertebral disk are included.

HIP *ARTHROPLASTY* (TOTAL HIP JOINT REPLACEMENT)

The hip joint is a ball and socket joint. The spherical head of the *femur* (the thigh bone) moves in the bony cup on the lower aspect of the bony pelvis (known as the *acetabulum*). The head of the femur is attached to the shaft by a narrowed portion called the neck of the femur, set at an angle to the shaft.

The operation of choice for severe, disabling arthritis of the hip, when it cannot be managed adequately by lesser methods, is total joint replacement. It consists of removing the head and neck of the femur and substituting an artificial head and neck with a special projection which is jammed down into the marrow cavity. The acetabulum is reamed out and an artificial joint-cup is fitted in place. Both of these prostheses are made of a nonreactive metal alloy and fixed by a special acrylic glue.

Complications

- Operative Hemorrhage
  This may be quite severe (in view of the extensive nature of the surgery) and require blood transfusion.

94   Informed Consent to Surgery

- Infection
  This is a disastrous event and every effort must be made to make the operating room comply with the very highest standards of aseptic precautions (because the exposed bone and joint are extremely vulnerable to infective bacteria).
- Dislocation of the Prosthesis
  This may occur with incorrect positioning of the lower limb following surgery.
- Late Displacement of the Prosthesis
  This is due to loosening inside the marrow cavity.
- Thrombosis and Embolism
  These must always be considered and guarded against in this type of surgery.
- Surgical Shock, Cardiac Failure, and Respiratory problems. These are quite common, since many of these patients are both elderly and debilitated.

A similar operation, but without replacement of the hip socket, is now—with increasing frequency—the operation of choice in fractures of the upper neck of the femur, and carries similar complications.

OPERATION FOR *HERNIATED INTERVERTEBRAL DISK*

This condition is also known as a displaced or protruded disk. The commonest level is the lowest lumbar region, where herniation produces the severe pain of sciatica and sometimes footdrop.

The operation, which is reserved for those cases not improved by nonsurgical measures, consists of removing a small portion of bone from the back of the vertebra, visualizing the herniated disk, and removing it. Sometimes a spinal fusion is included in the procedure.

Complications

- Injury to the Spinal Nerve
  This may produce pain, numbness, or paralysis. It occurs when the spinal nerve at the disk level is damaged at surgery.

- Injury to the Back of the Aorta
This results in catastrophic hemorrhage. It is a rare complication that occurs when the instrument which extracts the disk inadvertently tears the back of the aorta.
- Failure to Relieve the Symptoms, or Recurrence of Symptoms. This occurs when the operation fails to relieve pressure on the spinal nerve.

Conclusions and the Author's Personal Note

Once again, the reader is reminded that the overall mortality rate and complication rate in operative surgery is extremely low and getting progressively lower.

When I was commencing my surgical career, it seemed that none of my patients wanted to know very much about the proposed surgery and even less about the possible complications. Their attitude was very much along the lines of "You're my surgeon, you know what's best for me, and I trust you completely."

Happily, this was still very much the case when I retired after fifty years as a community surgeon, but with younger and more educated patients, with books on medical subjects and medical articles in newspapers and lay magazines, with radio and TV coverage of health care and—above all—with increasing medical litigation, there is a growing demand by patients for more detailed information.

One of the strongest newspaper articles on the subject of informed consent was written by the well-known medical writer, Dr. W. Gifford-Jones (pen name), and was entitled "How informed should a patient's consent to surgery be?" In it, he argues against the dangers of worrying the patient unnecessarily about the possibility of death or about complications that may never occur. He expresses concern about legislation that would force the doctor to relate all the hazards of treatment and, if that day ever comes, he says he hopes his first patient will be a politician. (I would have thought he'd choose a lawyer!) "He'll wonder," says Gifford-Jones, "why the doctor is becoming so fatigued as he recites the long list of complications that might, just might occur."

Emotionally, I might agree with everything that was said in the article about the hazards often outweighing the advantages of informed consent, about the usually inexact nature of the information given and received, and its unreliable comprehension and retention by the patient. Some of the best anesthetists I know have confided in me that they never give their patients the full information required for informed consent, and one of the best orthopedic surgeons I know, who does a great deal of hip surgery on very high-risk elderly patients, gave me the same confession.

But times are changing, and the modern patient, encouraged by lawyers and politicians, is becoming more demanding about full medical disclosure even if it means "knowing the worst."

I have witnessed a new generation of doctors spending an increasing amount of time discussing proposed lines of treatment and alternatives, as well as some of the complications, often to enthralled family audiences in the hospital corridors. Impressive as this may be, one wonders how much is understood and retained, or whether some important complication may have been inadvertently omitted.

At a surgical meeting in Toronto, a few years ago, I presented certain "Catch 22" medicolegal aspects of informed consent, with the patient and surgeon respectively on the witness stand, and postulated four possible scenarios:

In the first, the patient had been given all the requisite information prior to surgery but had genuinely forgotten.

In the second, the patient had been given all the requisite information but "chose to forget."

In the third, the surgeon failed to give all the requisite information but has genuinely forgotten.

In the fourth, the surgeon failed to give the requisite information but "chose to forget."

My question to those at the head table was "How does the court decide who is telling the truth?" In the absence of a convincing reply, I decided that this book must eventually be written.

Legal authorities have now declared that as long as the doctor writes down in his notes—at the time—that he has informed the patient preoperatively, the doctor's version will be accepted by the courts. In my opinion, such a decision is weighted against the patient, and this book seeks to provide a remedy to that situation and to be fair to both parties.

The decision to read any part or all of this book is up to the surgical patient's inclination and wishes, but at least all the most necessary information is available, and further questions can be directed to the patient's surgeon and personal physician.

The contents of this small volume should provide a safeguard both for you, the patient, and for the surgeon who will perform your operation.

Glossary of Medical Terms

A

ABDOMINOPERINEAL RESECTION Removal of the rectum and anal canal along with a portion of the colon.
ABLATE To remove or excise.
ACETABULUM The cup-like bony element of the hip joint which receives the ball of the femur, permitting free rotation.
ACHALASIA OF THE CARDIA Failure of the lower end of the gullet to relax, thus producing a chronic holdup of food and liquid and leading to a progressive dilatation of the gullet. This condition results in progressive malnutrition of the patient.
ACTINOMYCOSIS A fungal infection, occurring most commonly in the proximal portion of the colon and in the lungs.
ACUTE Sudden or of extremely rapid onset.
ADENOMA A benign (noncancerous) tumour.
ADHESION The sticking together of two organs or layers of tissue as a result of the fibrous healing process following inflammation.
AEROBIC Bacteria and other microorganisms which thrive in the presence of oxygen.
ALVEOLUS Sometimes known as Acinus. This is a minute sac lined by specialized cells such as those in the lungs.
ANAEROBIC Bacteria and other micro-organisms which thrive in the absence of oxygen.
ANAL CANAL The terminal portion of the digestive tract, between the rectum and the anal orifice.

ANAPHYLAXIS   An extremely dangerous degree of allergic response to foreign materials.

ANASTOMOSIS   The joining together of two structures, such as stomach to intestine or artery to graft.

ANEURYSM   A balloon-like dilatation of a blood vessel, e.g. an abdominal aortic aneurysm.

ANTERIOR RESECTION   Removal of the sigmoid colon (or more of the left colon) along with the rectum, but with anastomosis of the colon to the anal canal.

ANTICOAGULANT   A chemical which interferes with the normal blood-clotting mechanism.

AORTA   The main artery of the body, which carries oxygenated blood from the left side of the heart to the rest of the body, through its numerous branches.

ARDS   This is an abbreviation for the Acute Respiratory Distress Syndrome. In recent years it has been called the "Adult" Respiratory Distress Syndrome to distinguish it from the respiratory distress syndrome of the newborn. The adult condition, sometimes called **shock lung**, may follow severe trauma, severe sepsis, over-infusion of fluids or excessive transfusion of blood.

ARRHYTHMIA   Irregular rhythm, as in cardiac arrhythmia.

ARTERIOSCLEROSIS   Hardening of the arteries, usually due to atheromatous deposits, which sometimes become calcified.

ARTHROPLASTY   Surgical repair of a joint, as in total hip-joint replacement.

ASD   Abbreviation for arteriosclerosis or ateroslerosis.

ASPIRATION   Inhalation of contents other than gases, as in **aspiration pneumonia**, which results from the inhalation of stomach contents which have been vomited or regurgitated.

ATELECTASIS   Failure to expand, as in the lung (**pulmonary atelectasis**, partial or total).

ATHEROMA   A fatty substance which is deposited on the inner wall of arteries and causes their obstruction or ballooning.

ATHEROSCLEROSIS   Another name for arteriosclerosis.

ATRIUM   Usually refers to one of the upper chambers of the heart.

AXILLA   The armpit; a pyramidal space between the inner side of the upper arm and the upper rib cage, the collar bone (**clavicle**) and pectoral muscles in front, and the shoulder blade (**scapula**) with its attached muscles behind. It contains the bloodvessels and nerve trunks to the upper limb, lymph nodes and lymph vessels, as well as a varying amount of fat.

B

BACTEREMIA The presence of bacteria in the blood.

BENIGN Innocent, as in a benign (non-cancerous) tumour.

BILE A thick green fluid containing pigments from broken-down red blood cells, and bile salts which help in the digestion of fats. BILIARY SYSTEM This includes the liver which produces the bile, the gallbladder which stores and concentrates the bile, and the various bile ducts, ultimately terminating in the first part of the small intestine (**duodenum**).

BRONCHUS (pl. Bronchi) A breathing-tube which arises as a division of the windpipe. Each divides, in turn, into smaller tubes known as **bronchioles**.

BUERGER'S DISEASE A spastic condition of the blood-vessels, commonest in relatively young men who are heavy cigarette smokers, and in which portions of the limbs may be lost due to impaired blood supply.

BYPASS A technique for going around an obstruction, as in the gastrointestinal tract or the arterial system.

C

CANNULA A short stiff tube, usually inserted into a rubber or plastic tube as a connecting device.

CAPSULE A layer of tissue surrounding an organ and acting as an envelope, as in **thyroid capsule** or **prostatic capsule**.

CECUM The very first part of the large bowel, forming a pouch below the entrance of the small intestine, and is the area from which the appendix originates.

CECOSTOMY Usually tube cecostomy, the temporary suturing of a tube into the cecum as a "blow-off" device to complement a left-sided colon resection, in the absence of bowel obstruction.

CAPILLARY Usually refers to the very finest blood vessels between the smallest arteries and the smallest veins.

CARDIAC ARREST Sudden cessation of a detectable heart beat.

CARDIOGENIC SHOCK A state of circulatory collapse which results from a failure of the heart's action rather than such factors as sepsis or massive blood loss.

CARDIOPULMONARY BYPASS A system for circulating oxygenated blood through the body, not through the heart and lungs but through a special apparatus known as a pump-oxygenator. This makes it possible to operate on the heart without massive loss of blood.

CARDIOVASCULAR Pertaining to the circulation in the heart and blood-vessels.
CAROTID ARTERY The main artery to the head, (brain and face).
CATASTROPHIC Life-threatening, such as overwhelming infection or massive loss of blood.
CATHETER A tube (rubber or plastic) used to empty a fluid collection in a hollow organ such as the urinary bladder.
CELLULITIS A solid form of inflammation, without pus-formation.
CENTRAL VEIN A major vein which is in close proximity to the heart.
CHOLECYSTECTOMY Removal of the gallbladder, usually for stones.
COLON The large intestine, beyond the junction of the small intestine and the cecum. The ascending colon is on the right side of the abdomen, the transverse colon goes from right to left, the descending colon is on the left side, and the sigmoid colon is in the pelvis where it empties into the rectum.
COLOSTOMY A surgical opening of the colon onto the surface skin, with the feces emptying into a collection device. May be temporary or permanent.
COMMON BILE DUCT The bile duct formed by the junction of the hepatic duct and the cystic duct.
CONGENITAL A condition with which one is born, but not necessarily inherited.
CONSERVATIVE When applied to a surgical operation, it means one of less severity, in contrast to one of greater scope for the same condition. For example, **lumpectomy** rather than mastectomy for breast cancer.
CONSTRICTION Sometimes called a stricture, a narrowing which can produce some degree of obstruction.
CORONARY ARTERY One of the arteries supplying the heart's muscle.
CPR An abbreviation for Cardiopulmonary Resuscitation, which consists in obtaining an adequate airway, administering artificial respiration and applying external cardiac massage.
CREPITANT Usually refers to the presence of gas bubbles in the tissues, as in crepitant cellulitis.
CROHN'S DISEASE A chronic inflammatory condition of the digestive tract, commonest in the terminal small bowel and the colon.
CYST A balloon-like structure containing fluid and usually caused by obstruction to the outflow of a gland. A **pseudocyst** is formed by the accumulation of fluid next to a glandular structure such as the pancreas, and becomes surrounded by an enclosing sheet of tissue.
CYSTECTOMY Removal of the urinary bladder, usually for invasive

cancer, and combined with a procedure to divert the flow of urine.
CYSTIC DUCT The duct from the gallbladder to the common bile duct.
CYSTOSCOPE A telescopic instrument for viewing the interior of the urinary bladder.

D

DEHISCENCE Usually refers to the full-thickness disruption (opening up) of a recent surgical wound (as in a **burst abdomen**).
DEVASCULARIZED A structure which has lost its blood vessels or blood supply.
DIAPHRAGM The muscular sheet which separates the thoracic cavity from the abdominal cavity, and which plays a major role in respiration.
DISSECTION This term, when applied to arteries, refers to fragmentation of the blood vessel's lining, with the bloodstream finding new channels outside the main lumen.
DIVERTICULUM A pouch-like protrusion of the wall of a hollow structure. It may be solitary, as in the pharynx, or multiple, as in the colon. If it becomes inflamed, the condition (commonest in the colon) is called diverticulitis.
DORSAL This term is used to define a location on the back of the body. It is also used as a synonym for **thoracic**.
DRAINAGE As a surgical term, it refers to the provision of an outlet from a body cavity, for the escape of blood, bile, pus, or other fluids to the exterior. This may be done with various types of tubes, or simple strips of rubber. Drainage is the most important single element in the management of abscesses anywhere in the body.
DUMPING SYNDROME A possible complicating sequel of gastric surgery, due to rapid emptying of stomach contents into the small intestine. Characterized by faintness, sweating, nausea and palpitations after meals. Commoner after the Billroth 2 type of partial gastrectomy.
DUODENUM The first part of the small intestine and the area most vulnerable to so-called "stomach ulcers."

E

EDEMA The accumulation of fluid in the soft tissue spaces.
ELECTROLYTE A substance such as sodium, potassium, chloride, or bicarbonate, that breaks into electrically charged ions in solution.
EMBOLISM The release of blood clots into the circulation.
EMBOLUS A blood clot which has become detached from the interior of a vein and travels to a distant spot, where it lodges.

EMPHYSEMA   A lung disease in which there is a breakdown of the air-sacs. It is also a term for air in the tissue spaces, as in **subcutaneous emphysema** or **mediastinal emphysema**.

EMPYEMA   This term usually means an empyema of the chest cavity, and refers to an abscess of that cavity, but outside the lungs.

ENDARTERECTOMY   An operation in which a blocked artery is opened and the obstructing material is removed, in order to restore the blood flow from the open channel above to the open channel below.

ENDOTRACHEAL   Inside the windpipe. Usually refers to the tube which is inserted in the trachea for anesthesia or to obtain adequate respiration.

EPIDURAL ANESTHESIA   Similar to spinal anesthesia, but the main fluid channel is not entered.

EPIGASTRIC   The upper part of the belly, between the breastbone and the navel.

EPIGLOTTIS   A flap-like structure behind the tongue, which closes over the top of the larynx during swallowing.

ESOPHAGUS   The gullet, extending from the pharynx above to the stomach below, which it enters at a point known as the **cardia**.

EVISCERATION   The escape of intestine or other abdominal contents through a break in the wound.

F

FAILURE   This term is used mostly in connection with vital functions, e.g. cardiac, respiratory, hepatic or renal failure, and means a breakdown of the normal function.

FEMUR   The thigh-bone. The adjective is **femoral**, pertaining to the thigh, as in **femoral hernia** or **femoropopliteal bypass**.

FIBROSIS   A build-up of fibrous tissue, as in scarring. This is an essential mechanism in the healing process.

FISSURE   A crack in skin or mucous membrane, as in **anal fissure**.

FISTULA   An abnormal channel between the interior of a hollow organ and either the surface skin or the interior of another organ or body cavity, e.g. **bronchopleural**, **biliary**, or **anal fistula**.

G

GANGRENE   Death of a body part with some degree of putrefaction, usually as a result of deficient blood supply.

GASTRECTOMY   Partial or total. In the **Billroth 1 procedure**, the gastric stump is anastomosed to the duodenum; in the **Billroth 2 procedure**, it is anastomosed to the jejunum.

GASTROSTOMY Usually a temporary tube gastrostomy, used in abdominal surgery, in which stomach drainage (or feeding) is conducted by way of a tube which has been sutured into the stomach interior.
GOITRE An enlargement of the thyroid gland, which produces the hormone **thyroxin**, one which controls metabolism.
GRAVE'S DISEASE An extreme form of hyperthyroidism.

H
HALOTHANE An inhalation anesthetic used to produce general anesthesia.
HEMATOMA A collection of blood in a tissue space, either fluid or clotted.
HEMOLYSIS The breakdown of red cells in the blood, with release and then breakdown of **hemoglobin** (the oxygen-carrying pigment in the red cells).
HEMORRHOIDECTOMY Removal of anal piles.
HEMOSTAT An instrument designed to seize a bleeding point—during an operation—so that it can be dealt with by the application of a ligature or sealed by crushing.
HEMOTHORAX The presence of blood in the thoracic (pleural) cavity outside the lungs.
HEART BLOCK A condition in which only a portion of the heart-beats are transmitted from one chamber to another, due to a conduction defect.
HELLER OPERATION This is a procedure for the cure of achalasia of the cardia. Its main element is the vertical division of circular muscle fibres at the lower end of the esophagus (gullet).
HEPATIC Pertaining to the liver. (Subhepatic means under the liver, as in **subhepatic hematoma**).
HEPATORENAL SYNDROME Combined failure of the liver and kidneys.
HERNIA Commonly known as a "rupture." An abdominal hernia is an abnormal protrusion of peritoneum, in the form of a **hernial sac**, through a defect in the abdominal wall, either congenital or acquired.
HERNIATED DISK This is a protrusion of an intervertebral disk, i.e. one between two vertebral bodies, and is commonest in the lowest part of the spine.
HIATUS HERNIA A protrusion of the upper part of the stomach into the lower chest via an enlarged esophageal hiatus (the opening in the diaphragm through which the esophagus enters the abdomen). Some of these hernias are associated with reflux esophagitis.
HIRSCHSPRUNG'S DISEASE Congenital enlargement of the colon in in-

fants and children, caused by absence of essential nerve cells in the terminal portion of the large bowel and producing severe constipation and abdominal distension.

HORNER'S SYNDROME A condition caused by damage to the **sympathetic** nerve chain in the lower part of the neck. It produces a constriction of the pupil, a sinking back of the eyeball, a drooping of the upper eyelid, and a dryness and flushing of the face—all these on the affected side.

HYDROCELE A condition in which fluid accumulates in the protective sac around the testicle and may form a large swelling in the scrotum.

HYPERTENSION Raised blood pressure.

HYPERTROPHY Excessive growth of an organ or body-part.

HYPOVOLEMIC A state of lowered blood volume, as in surgical shock secondary to severe hemorrhage, or massive burns.

I

ILEAL Pertaining to the ileum. An **ileal loop** is a segmemt of ileum with its intact blood-supply, mainly used for implantation of the ureter. An **ileal pouch** is a surgically constructed pouch between the end of the ileum and the body surface, with a valvular orifice so that the patient can empty the pouch by catheter.

ILEOSTOMY An artificial opening of the terminal small intestine (the ileum) onto the surface, where it discharges its contents into a special waterproof collecting device.

ILEUM The third and major portion of the small intestine, between the jejunum above and the cecum below.

ILIAC This term refers to major bloodvessels in the pelvis and to a portion of the bony pelvis.

IMMUNOSUPPRESSIVE A term for chemicals, viruses, radiation, or other factors which interfere with the action of the immune system.

IMPERFORATE Absence of the normal opening, as in **imperforate anus**, a congenital absence of the anal orifice or anal canal.

INCISIONAL HERNIA A hernia which occurs at the site of a previous surgical incision, due to disruption of the abdominal muscle structures beneath the scar.

INCOMPETENCE A term usually applied to one-way valves in the body that are no longer functioning properly, as in **venous incompetence**.

INCONTINENCE A failure to contain urine or feces in the normal fashion, with involuntary leakage of these excretions.

INFERIOR VENA CAVA The principal vein to that part of the body which is below the level of the heart.

INFILTRATION Invasion or diffusion of soft tissue spaces by material not found normally in that tissue, such as cancer or fat. Also a term for local anesthetic injection into soft tissues.
INFUSION The introduction of fluid into blood vessels or soft tissues, as in intravenous or subcutaneous infusion.
INGUINAL Pertaining to the groin region, as in **inguinal hernia**.
INTRACRANIAL Inside the cranium, which is the upper part of the skull, above the facial bones.
INTUSSUSCEPTION The telescoping of a segment of bowel into the adjoining segment of bowel in a progressive fashion.
IRREDUCIBLE Generally refers to an inability to push back a hernial protrusion (or prolapse) by gentle pressure, or by having the patient lie down.
ISLET CELLS The cells in the pancreas that produce insulin and other hormones of metabolism.
ISTHMUS A narrow connecting portion, as in **thyroid isthmus**.

J
JAUNDICE A yellow discolouration of the eyes and skin, sometimes progressing to green and brown, due to the presence of bile pigments in the tissues—where they are deposited from an excess in the blood.
JEJUNOSTOMY The surgical insertion of a tube into the jejunum for the purpose of introducing nutritional fluids where food cannot be taken in the normal fashion.
JEJUNUM The second part of the small intestine, between the duodenum—from which it receives bile and pancreatic juice—and the ileum, into which it empties.

K
KELOID A hard, raised scar, with a tendency to recur after excision. It is commonest after burns and in genetically susceptible individuals.

L
LAPAROTOMY Operative entry into the abdomen, usually for exploratory purposes. Increasingly replaced by modern scanning techniques.
LARYNX The voice box, containing the vocal cords.
LUMBAR A descriptive term for the lower back. The lumbar spine consists of five vertebrae below the thoracic spine, and forms the firm back support to the abdomen and pelvis.
LUMPECTOMY The surgical removal of a lump. As a method of dealing

with very early breast cancer it has gained in popularity over the past decade, combined with chemotherapy or radiation, and combined with exploration of the axillary lymph nodes.
LYMPHATIC SYSTEM This is the third circulation, other than arteries and veins, and consists of lymphatic vessels, lymph nodes (glands), and lymph channels. They contain lymph, a thin fluid similar to plasma.

M
MALIGNANT HYPERTHERMIA A rare and grave complication of general anesthesia, characterized by very high fever and muscular rigidity. A familial history of this disorder serves as a warning to the anesthetist, since a tendency to this condition is inherited.
MASTECTOMY An operation in which the breast is removed.
MECKEL'S DIVERTICULUM A congenital tubular pouch in the last 2 feet of the ileum, like an extra appendix, and found in 2 percent of the population. It may become acutely inflamed or bleed from an ulcer that resembles a stomach ulcer. In either event it may perforate if not removed surgically.
MECONIUM A thick, glue-like material present in the intestines of the newborn infant, prior to its replacement by feces. If it becomes so thick as to cause a bowel obstruction, the condition is known as **meconium ileus**.
MEDIASTINUM This is the term for the space that contains all the anatomical structures in the chest that are between the two lungs, and are outside the pleural cavities. It includes the heart and great blood vessels, the trachea, esophagus, and numerous lymph nodes, as well as other tissues and structures. An inflammation of the soft tissues in the mediastinum is known as **mediastinitis** and is extremely serious.
MENINGES The coverings of the brain and spinal cord. The outer covering, which is tough and fibrous, is known as the **dura**. The inner layer, which is thin and delicate, is known as the **arachnoid**. It encloses the fluid which circulates around the brain and spinal cord, the **cerebrospinal fluid**. Infection of this space is known as **meningitis**.
MESENTERY The double sheet of peritoneum from which the stomach and intestines, as well as their appendages, are suspended, and which contain the blood vessels, the nerves, lymphatics and lymph-nodes of these organs. Thrombosis of these vessels is known as **mesenteric thrombosis**, and embolism to these vessels is known as **mesenteric embolism**, in which a clot (usually from the heart) lodges in a mesenteric artery, shutting off the blood-supply to the organ.

MOBILIZATION   The freeing up of separated structures so that they may be joined together without undue tension.
MYOCARDIAL INFARCTION   Death of heart muscle due to blockage of the blood supply to the heart.
MYOGLOBIN   The pigmented complex protein in muscle, that is the equivalent of hemoglobin.
MYXEDEMA   An extreme form of thyroxin deficiency.

N
NASOGASTRIC TUBE   A tube, either rubber or plastic, inserted via the nose into the stomach, for gastric drainage or for the introduction of nutritional fluids where food cannot be taken normally.
NECROSIS   Death of tissues or cells.
NEPHRECTOMY   Removal of the kidney.
NEURALGIA   Pain along the distribution of a sensory nerve.
NEUROMA   A swelling on the cut end of a nerve, or a true tumour of nerve tissue—one which is benign.
NEUROTOXIN   Nerve poison. Aside from such man-made poisons as those for chemical warfare, certain bacteria are capable of producing their own highly potent nerve toxins. A prime example is the bacterium that causes tetanus.

O
OCCLUSION   The blocking up of a hollow tube or orifice. Most often used in connection with arterial obstruction, e.g. coronary occlusion.
ORTHOPEDIC   Pertaining to surgery of the skeletal system.
OSTOMY   A term for any surgically produced, artificial opening, such as a colostomy or ileostomy.
OXYGENATION   The supply of oxygen to cells, tissues or organs.

P
PALLIATIVE   Usually refers to a mode of treatment that relieves the unpleasant symptoms of a disease rather than curing the condition. It is directed to improving the quality rather than the duration of life.
PANCREAS   The sweetbread. A glandular organ, situated behind the stomach, that produces powerful digestive fluids, which it discharges into the duodenum. It also produces insulin, which it releases into the blood stream for the control of sugar metabolism. A severe inflammation of the pancreas is known as **acute pancreatitis**.
PARATHYROIDS   A group of small glands situated behind the thyroid gland, on both sides of the neck, and essential for the metabolism of

calcium compounds throughout the body.

PAROTITIS Inflammation of the salivary gland in front of the ear, called the **parotid**. The common form is known as mumps. The dangerous form, which may follow any operation, is known as acute parotitis.

PENETRATING A term applied to a condition such as an ulcer which burrows into an adjacent organ to which it is adherent.

PERFORATED A term applied to such conditions as appendicitis, gastric or duodenal ulcer, and diverticulitis of the colon, when a localized hole occurs in the wall of a hollow organ, resulting in the escape of the contents ino a body cavity and producing such problems as peritonitis.

PERFUSION The circulation of blood or other fluids through the blood vessels of a specific organ. An example is the perfusion of blood in the muscular walls of the heart via the coronary arterial system.

PERICARDIUM The smooth membranous envelope that completely surrounds the heart and related great blood vessels.

PERINEUM (Adj. Perineal) The area between the vulva or scrotum in front and the anal ring behind.

PERIPHERAL VEIN In contrast to a central vein, this is usually in the upper or lower limb; sometimes a superficial vein of the neck.

PERITONEUM The thin membrane that lines the abdominal cavity, extends onto the mesenteries and covers most of the abdominal organs. The term **acute peritonitis** is used for a rapidly occurring and dangerous inflammation of the peritoneal cavity and usually results from an acutely inflamed abdominal organ, especially one that has perforated.

PHARYNX The cavity between the nostrils and mouth above and the esophagus below.

PILONIDAL SINUS A discharging channel in the tailbone region, caused by ingrown tufts of hair. If blocked, it may form a pilonidal abscess.

PLAQUE Other than its dental application this term usually refers to a deposit of atheroma on the inner lining of an artery.

PLEURA The thin sheet that lines the chest cavities and covers the lungs.

PNEUMOTHORAX The presence of air in the thoracic (pleural) cavity outside the lungs, either by external injury or by leakage from a weakened or diseased area of the lung.

POLYP A spheroidal tumour, often small and multiple, as in the condition known as **polyposis**. Polypi may be benign or malignant.

PROLAPSE A term used to descibe the protrusion of a body part beyond its normal confines, as in prolapsing hemorrhoids, where the anal piles protrude well beyond the anal orifice.

PROSTATECTOMY   Removal of the prostate gland.
PROSTHESIS   An artificial device inserted into or attached to the body, such as an artificial limb.
PULMONARY   Pertaining to the lungs, as in **pulmonary embolism** or **pulmonary edema**.
PYLEPHLEBITIS   Sometimes known as **portal pyemia**. A septic embolism to the liver, causing liver abscesses.
PYLORUS   The outlet of the stomach, where it joins the duodenum.

R

RADICAL   Usually refers to a more severe or major type of procedure, in contrast to a lesser (conservative) procedure for the same condition, such as performing a lumpectomy for breast cancer rather than a lumpectomy.
RAMSTEDT OPERATION   Division of the pyloric sphincter for congenital hypertrophic pyloric stenosis.
RAYNAUD'S DISEASE   A spastic disease of the arteries, commoner in young women, characterized by an extreme sensitivity of the small blood vessels in the skin to cold temperatures.
RECTUM   That portion of the large bowel between the sigmoid colon above and the anal canal below.
REDUCIBLE   Usually refers to a hernial protrusion (or prolapse) that can be pushed back by gentle pressure or by the patient lying down.
REFLUX   Regurgitation, as in esophageal reflux.
REFLUX ESOPHAGITIS   Inflammation of the lower esophagus caused by the persistent regurgitation of acid stomach contents (sometimes by alkaline intestinal contents following gastric surgery).
RENAL   Pertaining to the kidney.
RESECTION   Excision or surgical removal.
RESECTOSCOPE   An instrument that provides telescopic viewing of the area in which a resection is being performed, as in a **transurethral prostatectomy** (TUR).
RESPIRATORY   Pertaining to the broad subject of breathing, and of gaseous exchange in the lungs, circulation, tissues and cells.
RETENTION   Containment, or failure to empty, as in **urinary retention**, in which the bladder fails to empty properly. May be partial or total.
RETRACTION   The opposite of prolapse. Withdrawal from the surface, such as the indrawing of a colostomy or ileostomy opening.
RETROPERITONEAL   Behind the peritoneal lining of the abdomen's back wall. The kidneys and ureters as well as the great vessels of the abdomen are retroperitoneal, as is the sympathetic nerve chain.

RETROPUBIC Behind the pubis. This term is usually applied to a type of prostatectomy in which the prostate gland is approached from ouside the bladder, in contrast to a **suprapubic** prostatectomy which is performed from inside the bladder.

S
SCLEROSANT A substance which causes inflammation, clotting and occlusion, as in the injection treatment of varicose veins.
SEPTIC Infected. Usually with pus formation.
SEPTICEMIA The proliferation of bacteria in the bloodstream.
SEROMA A collection of serum in the soft tissues.
SINUS A channel which communicates with the skin but not with the interior of an organ, e.g. a suture sinus or **pilonidal sinus**.
SKIN FLAP An area of skin, usually with some underlying fat, that is raised by the surgeon in order to cover any open area at the end of the operation.
SLIDING HERNIA A hernia in which the bowel or bladder forms part of the hernial sac wall, rather than simply the content of the sac.
SPERMATIC CORD The cord-like structure which carries blood vessels and nerves to the testicle and the vas deferens from the testicle.
SPHINCTER A muscular ring controlling the passage of contents in one organ or segment of a hollow organ into the next organ or segment, as in **anal sphincter**.
SPINAL ANESTHESIA A method in which an anesthetic drug is injected into the cerebrospinal fluid by puncturing the dura, in contrast to **epidural anesthesia** where the dura is not punctured.
SPLEEN The organ which lies to the left of the stomach and is concerned with the production of certain blood cells (other than red cells), and with the destruction of aging blood cells.
SPLENECTOMY Removal of the spleen.
STENOSIS Narrowing in a hollow structure, as in an artery.
STERNUM The breast bone. (**Substernal** or **retrosternal** means behind the sternum).
STOMA Another name for the opening of an ostomy.
STRICTURE Narrowing, usually by scarring. Constriction.
STRANGULATION This medical term refers to the shutting off of the blood supply to an organ.
SUBCUTANEOUS A term for the layer of tissue under the skin, mainly composed of fat and connective tissue.
SUBPHRENIC ABSCESS A closed collection of pus under the diaphragm.
SUPRAPUBIC The lower part of the belly between the navel and the

groins. This term is also used for a prostate removal done through the bladder.

SURGICAL SHOCK This is a state of circulatory collapse in which the blood pressure falls abruptly; it is associated with widespread organ failure and disruption of cell metabolism. The common varieties are **hypovolemic shock**, as in massive blood-loss, **cardiogenic shock**, as in acute coronary occlusion. and **septic shock** as in massive infections.

SYMBIOTIC GANGRENE A type of spreading soft tissue gangrene caused by two different types of bacteria that work in biological union. Their combined effect is much more destructive than that of either individual types of microorganism.

SYMPATHETIC NERVOUS SYSTEM A portion of the nervous system that is not under voluntary control and is involved in the contraction of muscle in the digestive tract, contraction of blood vessels, sweating, and other involuntary functions.

SYNDROME A characteristic combination of clinical symptoms and signs.

T

TETANUS Lockjaw. A highly fatal infection caused by a virulent anaerobic bacterium, which produces a potent neurotoxin and ultimately causes respiratory paralysis.

THORACIC Pertaining to the chest and its contents.

THORACIC OUTLET The apex of the axilla, through which pass the major blood vessels and nerve trunks to the upper limb.

THROMBOPHLEBITIS Usually called "phlebitis." Inflammation (and clotting) of a vein.

THYROID GLAND A glandular structure in the neck. It produces and circulates a hormone, **thyroxin**, which has a profound influence on the body's rate of metabolism. The condition of thyroxin excess is known as **hyperthyroidism** and the condition of thyroxin deficiency is known as **hypothyroidism**.

THYROIDECOMY Partial or complete removal of the thyroid gland.

THYROID STORM An extreme form of hyperthyroidism which may come on when thyroidectomy is performed for Grave's disease.

TISSUE An aggregation of cells of the same type, e.g. muscle, cartilage, nerve tissue. The term **soft tissues** refers mainly to fat and connective tissues that bind cell layers together, and **tissue spaces** refer to the spaces between cells and cell-layers.

TRACHEA The windpipe, connecting to the bronci and lungs.

TRACHEOSTOMY Sometimes called a **tracheotomy**. A surgical opening in the upper trachea, usually performed for laryngeal obstruction or to assist respiratory control in patients with a depressed breathing mechanism who are on machine assistance.

U
ULCERATIVE COLITIS   A severe inflammatory condition of the colon associated with widespread ulceration of that organ.
UMBILICAL   Pertaining to the navel.
UNDESCENDED TESTICLE   A testicle that has failed to reach its normal position in the scrotum. It is associated with diminished fertility and an increased tendency to testicular cancer.
URETER   The tube that carries urine from the kidney to the bladder.
URETEROSTOMY   An artificial opening of the ureter for the diversion of urine, as with removal of the bladder.
URETEROSIGMOIDOSTOMY   An anastomosis between the ureters and the sigmoid colon. (Also known as the Coffey Procedure).
URETHRA   The channel through which urine is passed from the bladder to the exterior.

V
VAGOTOMY   Division of the vagus nerves to the stomach.
VAGUS NERVES   Two nerves that supply the stomach and other organs with involuntary nerve fibres. They cause the production of highly acid gastric juice. They also control emptying via the pylorus.
VARICOSE VEINS   Dilated tortuous veins, usually superficial and visible. Mostly due to a breakdown of the valves in the veins.
VAS DEFERENS   The tube carrying semen from the testicle.
VASOSPASTIC   A condition of spasm and narrowing of the blood vessels, mainly affecting the smaller arteries.
VEIN GRAFT   A portion of vein (usually from the front of the thigh) that is used as a substitute for artery in arterial surgery.
VEIN STRIPPING   An operation for venous incompetence, in which the impaired vein is removed by means of a long instrument known as a vein stripper.
VENOUS   Pertaining to the veins.
VISCUS   (Pl. Viscera). Aother name for an organ.
VOLVULUS   Twisting of the bowel, eventually causing intestinal obstruction and blockage of the blood vessels.

W
WHIPPLE PROCEDURE   A radical operation for cancer of the pancreas or bile ducts.

ABOUT THE AUTHOR

Graduated January 1936 from the Middlesex Hospital (London University) with the degree of M.R.C.S.,L.R.C.P. (Gold Medallist in Surgery)

Other degrees:
1. M.B., B.S. London
2. F.R.C.S. England
3. F.R.C.S.C.

Former appointments:
1. Chief of Surgery, Dundurn Military Hospital, Saskatchewan, during World War 2.
2. Chief of Surgery, Royal Jubilee Hospital, Victoria, B.C.
3. President of the B.C. Surgical Society.
4. Chairman of the Section of General Surgery in the B.C. Medical Association.
5. Chief of Surgery, Algoma District Medical Group in Sault Ste. Marie, Ontario (now a 40 man group and growing).